DEDICATION

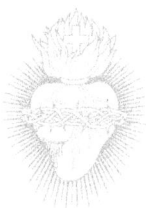

Sacred Heart of Jesus

NICOLE

Keith, thank you for growing closer to me as you grew closer to God

Evan and Charles, keep shining bright

*All those that encouraged me to imagine and believe,
especially my sister, parents and grandparents*

KATHRYN

*My husband and best friend, Mike, thank you for being
on this adventure with me!*

Sophia, Gabrielle, and Joseph, you bring me so much joy!

My parents, thank you for all the nurturing you gave me!

ISBN: 979-8-9933850-0-6 (paperback)
ISBN: 979-8-9933850-1-3 (ebook)

CONTENTS

Appendices

Nurturing
Whole
Health

You,
Your Baby
and God
in the
First Year

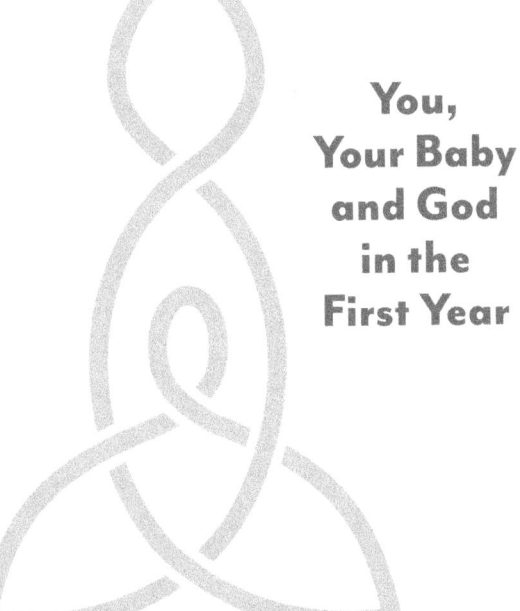

Nicole Lea, RN, CPNP and Kathryn Italia, MD

Hello Eema

ACKNOWLEDGMENTS

Dear friends such as Bao, Tam, and Karen, who encouraged me with nights of food and fellowship and helped me ground the dream in our Catholic faith.

Father Cascade for bold homilies at The Pines Catholic Camp. It is time to take the first step for F.A.M.I.L.Y. (Forget About Me, I Love You!).

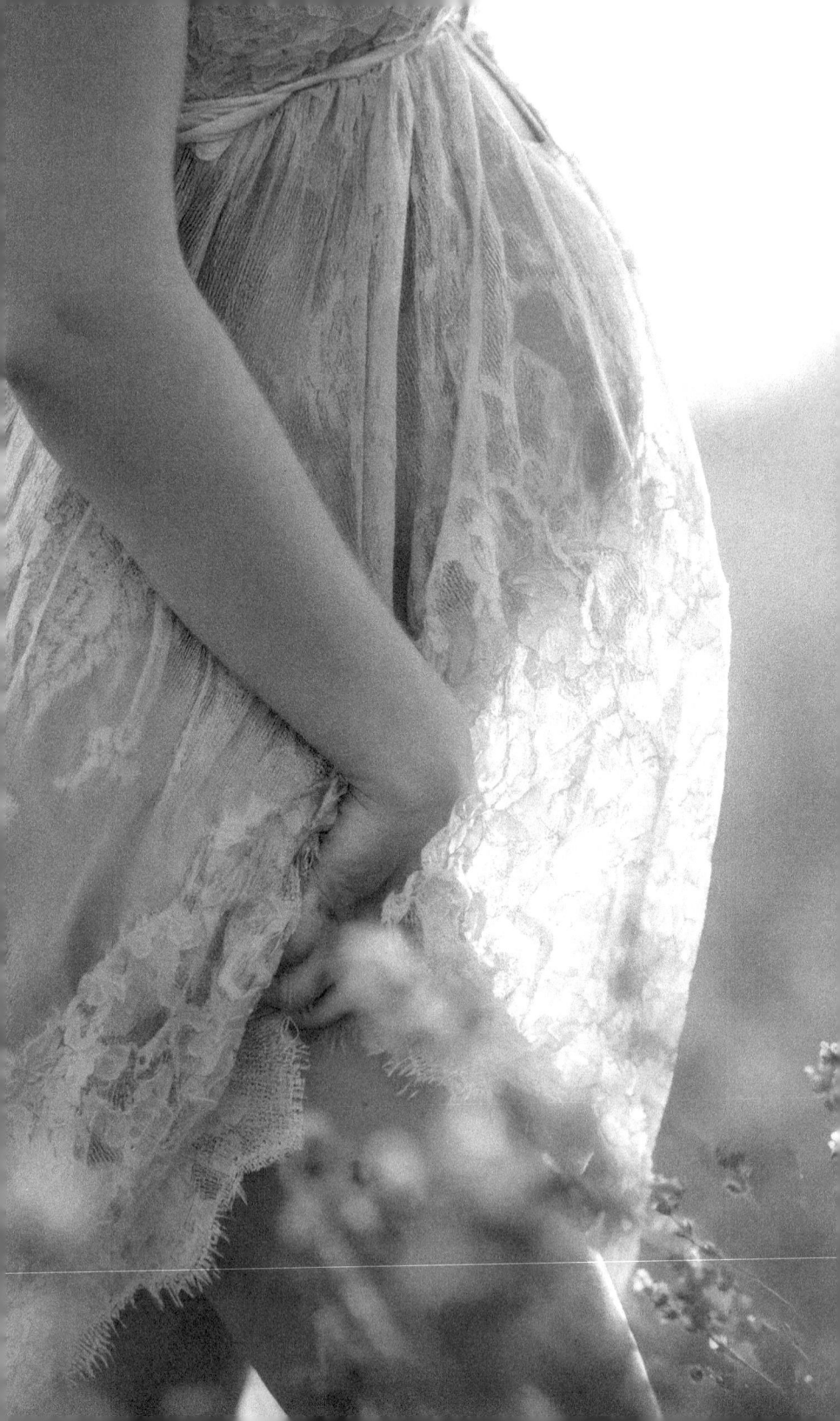

Introduction

"Beloved, we are God's children now;
what we shall be has not yet been revealed."

—1 John 3:2

Our ability to mother well begins with our relationship with God. He beckons us to boldly approach Him and abide in His presence, knowing that our hearts grow strong and confident only with Him at our side. Through this deepening relationship, we become the mothers our children need, women whose love for God shapes every aspect of their parenting.

As mothers, our ultimate goal is to raise our children to know and love God. This calling goes beyond world measures of success; our purpose is fixed on eternity. One day, we will stand before Him, and hopefully say, "Lord, I did everything I could to bring my children to You." When we embrace this eternal perspective, we can find peace even in life's imperfect, messy moments, knowing we are doing our best to draw our children to God.

"For God did not give us a spirit of cowardice
but rather of power and love and self-control."

—2 Timothy 1:7

As new moms, we are energized and excited to learn all there is to know to take the best care of our babies. We believe that when our faith is strong, we can better handle the physical, emotional, and mental demands of motherhood. This book guides you through nurturing all aspects of health for you and your baby, while keeping God at the center.

Above all, we pray this book helps you build a deep, personal relationship with God the Father, His Son, Jesus, and the Holy Spirit through prayer. This foundation of faith sustains us when life's distractions and hardships arise, giving us strength to persevere and hope to continue forward.

To help you on this journey, we'd like to share our own stories of how God has shaped our lives and brought us together to write this book.

Nicole's Story

I was raised in the Catholic Church, with deep roots in the faith tracing back through generations. On my mother's side, our Catholic heritage reaches back more than five hundred years to Germany, where a church still holds the graves of my ancestors. My father, originally not Catholic, converted when I was preparing for my Confirmation. As he sought answers to my many questions about faith, he found his own journey leading him to the Church.

Like many, I strayed in college, but ultimately, I found my way back. At twenty-six, I was married in the Catholic Church, but seven years later, my marriage ended. It was a painful chapter; one I will share with my children when the time is right. The marriage was later annulled, and for a few years, I found myself stepping away from the Catholic faith, searching for something to fill the void in my heart.

But God, in His relentless pursuit, never stopped calling me home. In His mercy, He led me back. When I married my now husband of ten years, we committed our marriage to Christ within the Church. Since then, our faith has been the cornerstone of our family. We are actively involved in multiple ministries and are beyond grateful for the grace that sustains us.

My perspective on life shifted when, at forty-three, I faced medical challenges that required a complete hysterectomy. What once felt like unbearable suffering I now see as a profound blessing. That season of pain stripped me of control, forcing me to surrender completely to God. And in that surrender, I found intimacy with my Lord and Savior like never before.

But the challenges didn't stop there. My career in nursing, with more than twenty years of caring for others across multiple specialties, took an unexpected turn. Despite my dedication, I faced struggles that shook my confidence and led to an unexpected career change. I was bitter, having wrapped my entire identity in being a healthcare professional.

Through this difficult season, God revealed a profound truth: I had placed my worth in my profession rather than in Him. It took stepping away from my work to realize that my primary identity isn't as a nurse, a wife, or even a mother; it is as a beloved daughter of God.

"Perhaps you were born for such a time as this."
—Esther 4:14

That realization didn't come easily. I wrestled with God, questioning why He would allow everything I worked for to unravel. But through my suffering, His presence became my constant companion. The more I leaned into Him, the stronger I became, until my identity was no longer defined by titles or roles, but by my relationship with God.

During my sabbatical from work as I healed, I volunteered at a women's pregnancy crisis center, teaching basic mothering skills, such as how to take a temperature, change a diaper, and practice safe sleep habits. As I worked with these women, I searched for a book that would help them cultivate their spiritual health with their physical and emotional well-being, something that acknowledged the profound connection between faith and motherhood.

But I couldn't find one.

The world talks a lot about physical, mental, and emotional health, but rarely about spiritual health. This is an essential part of the equation. When I searched for resources that spoke specifically to Catholic mothers, I found a gap. There wasn't a book that addressed the holistic needs of a mother raising children to be healthy in mind, body, heart, and spirit.

That's when I heard God whisper, *Why don't you write it?*

This book is the result of that call, a journey that has stretched and humbled me in ways I never expected. Just when I began to doubt, God's grace led Kathryn and I to meet at a Catholic women's conference! Our different paths gave us complementary perspectives on caring for mothers and children. After we met, it was clear the book must be completed and put into your hands.

Kathryn's Story

I grew up in a faith-filled household, and my journey with God began early. Throughout my college years, my faith increased as I became deeply involved in Catholic campus ministry. I served as an RCIA sponsor (now OCIA), participated in retreats, and eventually took on leadership roles. I left college feeling spiritually strong. During medical school and residency, I continued attending Mass weekly but found it increasingly difficult to stay involved in parish activities. Once my husband and I had children, we continued to attend Mass on Sundays and discuss our faith at home. Yet balancing work and family life was demanding, and I admit that my relationship with Christ often took a back seat.

In 2022 I had the opportunity to transition out of private practice pediatrics to stay home with my children. While I felt deeply blessed to be with them more, the shift initially left me questioning my identity. For more than fourteen years, I had defined myself as a physician. Who was I now? I wrestled with this question for several months. I joined a women's Bible study at my parish, spent hours at our parish's perpetual adoration chapel, and began using the Hallow app to pray. Ultimately, like Nicole, I realized that for years I had been defining myself by what I did or the roles I played. But this time of transformation finally made me realize whose I was. I am a child of God.

"For through faith you are all children of God in Christ Jesus."

—Galatians 3:26

As I rediscovered my identity in Christ, I also looked back on my career in medicine with a new perspective. From a young age, I knew I wanted to be a pediatrician. I easily recall summers with my brothers and cousins playing doctor, curing "patients" of such maladies as "cucamonga phobia" (as Cookie Monster once diagnosed Ernie having) or "silly-itis." It seemed so easy and fun back then. My cousin and I would give our patients little candies as medicine, and they would be magically cured!

Of course, practicing real medicine is significantly more complex than our simple childhood games. I looked forward to seeing my patients grow and following up with them year after year. Indeed, it was an honor and privilege to care for children of all ages and to help their families through the joys and challenges of parenting. However, as the years passed, I began noticing a deep sense of anxiety and uncertainty in many parents and the children and teens they brought in for care. Anxiety and depression were rising, and I often found myself spending more time discussing mental health than physical illness.

Something was missing. Where was God in all of this?

After leaving the daily practice of medicine and rediscovering my true identity in Christ, I searched for ways that I could impact those around me. I kept thinking about all those parents who seemed uncertain and all the children and teenagers who seemed lost. It became clear to me that helping others embrace their true identity in Christ might be the key to finding the joy, freedom, and security we all long for.

And then, as only could have been by God's design, my path crossed with Nicole's. I shared my story, and she shared her vision. I am incredibly blessed that she asked me to collaborate with her on this project.

A Note from Kathryn and Nicole

Throughout this book, you'll notice that most of the chapters are written in a first-person voice. When you come across personal reflections or anecdotes embedded directly in the main text, these represent Nicole's own journey and experiences. You'll also find a few personal insets written by Kathryn. While our individual voices appear in different ways, the entire book is the result of a true collaboration, drawing on both of our professional backgrounds, personal experiences, and shared desire to support mothers and babies in all aspects of health.

OUR PRAYER FOR YOU

"In you, O Lord, do I put my trust and
confidently take refuge; let me never
be put to shame or confusion!"

—Psalm 71:1

Our prayer for you is that this book blesses you. We pray it will help you build a solid foundation in Christ, guiding you to navigate the joys and challenges of parenting with confidence, clarity, and faith. That through it, you will come to know, with your entire being, the boundless love of God. May you experience the peace of Jesus and the power of the Holy Spirit who dwells within you.

Blessings,

Nicole and Kathryn

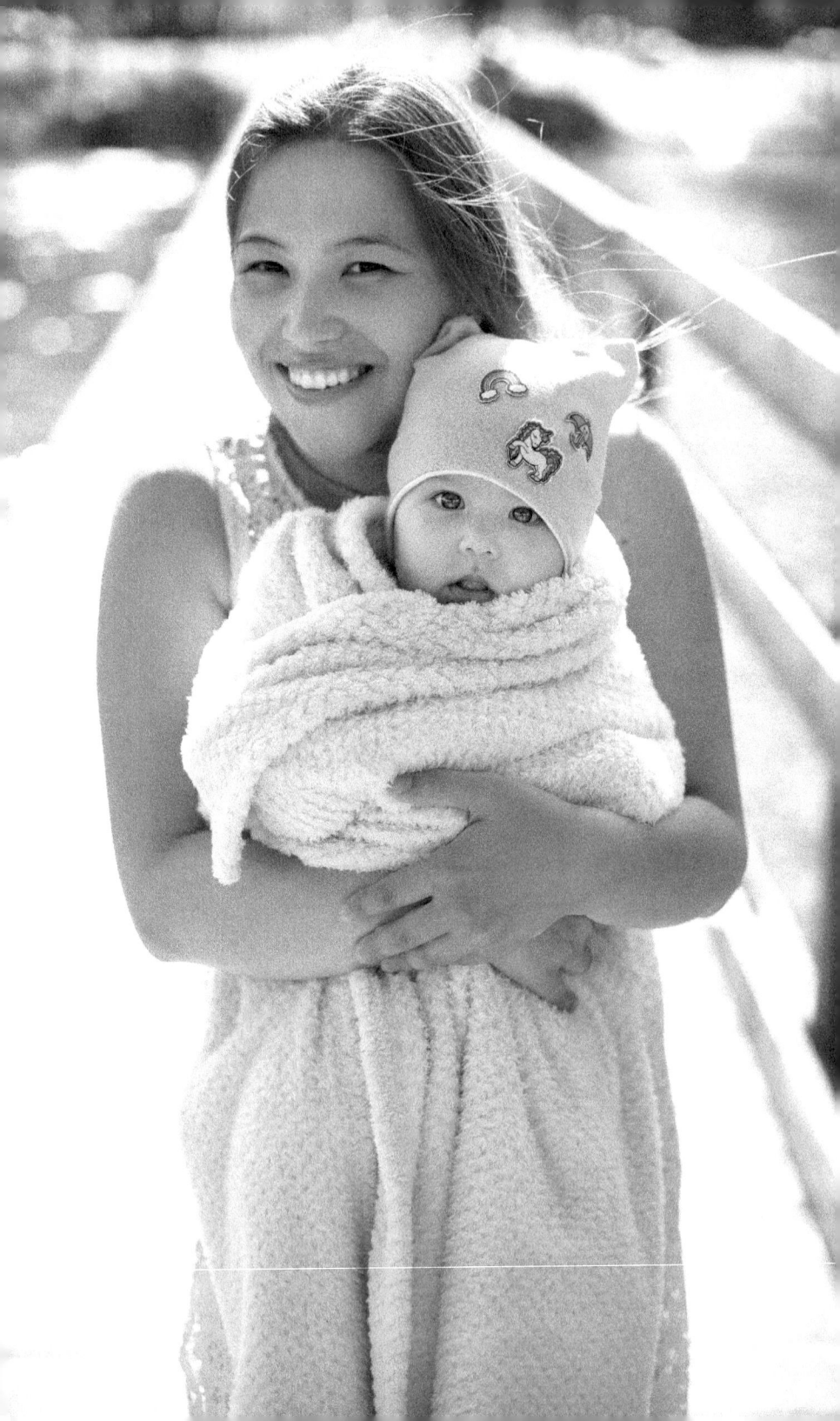

To All Our Mothers

Every journey to motherhood reflects God's unique plan. This book is written for all mothers who nurture and raise children, recognizing the diverse ways families come together. Know you are most welcomed here and your path to motherhood is equally profound and worthy of celebration.

> Love brought you to life as a family. Love sustains you through good and bad times. ... What you do in your family to create a community of love, to help each other to grow, and to serve those in need is critical, not only for your own sanctification but for the strength of society and our Church. It is a participation in the work of the Lord, a sharing in the mission of the Church. It is holy.[1]

God's call to motherhood takes many beautiful forms. For some, children are conceived through the sacred bond of marriage. Through this union, as the Church teaches, "Christ bestows on marriage and the family the grace necessary to witness to the love of God and to live the life of communion."[2] This divine plan connects the family to God's work from Creation to its final fulfillment in Christ.[3]

The beauty of God's plan for families can also extend beyond biological bonds. In adoption, many mothers answer God's call

---

1   United States Conference of Catholic Bishops, *Follow the Way of Love* (Washington, D.C.: USCCB, 1994), Accessed June 9, 2025, https://www.usccb.org/topics/marriage-and-family-life-ministries/follow-way-love.

2   Synod of Bishops, *Relatio Synodi: The Pastoral Challenges of the Family in the Context of Evangelization*, vatican.va, October 18, 2014, accessed June 11, 2025, https://www.vatican.va/roman_curia/synod/documents/rc_synod_doc_20141018_relatio-synodi-familia_en.html#The_Family_in_God's_Salvific_Plan.

3   Synod of Bishops, *Relatio Synodi*.

to protect and nurture His children, living out the sacred mission described in Scripture: "And the king will say to them in reply, 'Amen, I say to you, whatever you did for one of these least brothers of mine, you did for me'" (Matthew 25:40).

For our single mothers, we echo the bishops' words of solidarity from their document "Follow the Way": "To be faced with all the responsibilities of parenting by yourself is a challenge that touches the very core of your life."[4] Your strength in choosing life and creating a loving home is a testament to God's grace working through you.

No matter what your family situation might be, remember that "relationships and circumstances within your family may have changed, but God's love for you is ever-present and does not come to an end."[5]

Whether your motherhood story began with the sacrament of marriage, through adoption paperwork or single parenting, a hospital delivery room or an international journey, your experience is sacred. Your family, in whatever form God has blessed you with, forms a domestic church, nurturing faith and love in the next generation.

Though there may be some topics in this book that do not directly apply to every mother, the core message of nurturing whole health applies to all. Your journey may have unique challenges and joys, but you are an integral part of the motherhood community this book serves.

As you read these pages, please know that you belong here. Your motherhood journey, with all its challenges and victories, matters deeply. Whether your path to motherhood came through adoption, single parenthood, the traditional bonds of marriage, or another path, your story enriches our community of faith.

---

4   USCCB, *Follow the Way of Love*.

5   *Follow the Way of Love*.

"We know that all things work for good for those who love God, who are called according to his purpose."

—Romans 8:28

Your family reflects God's perfect design for bringing parents and children together. As you continue your journey of nurturing whole health for yourself and your child, may you find wisdom, encouragement, and support in the pages that follow.

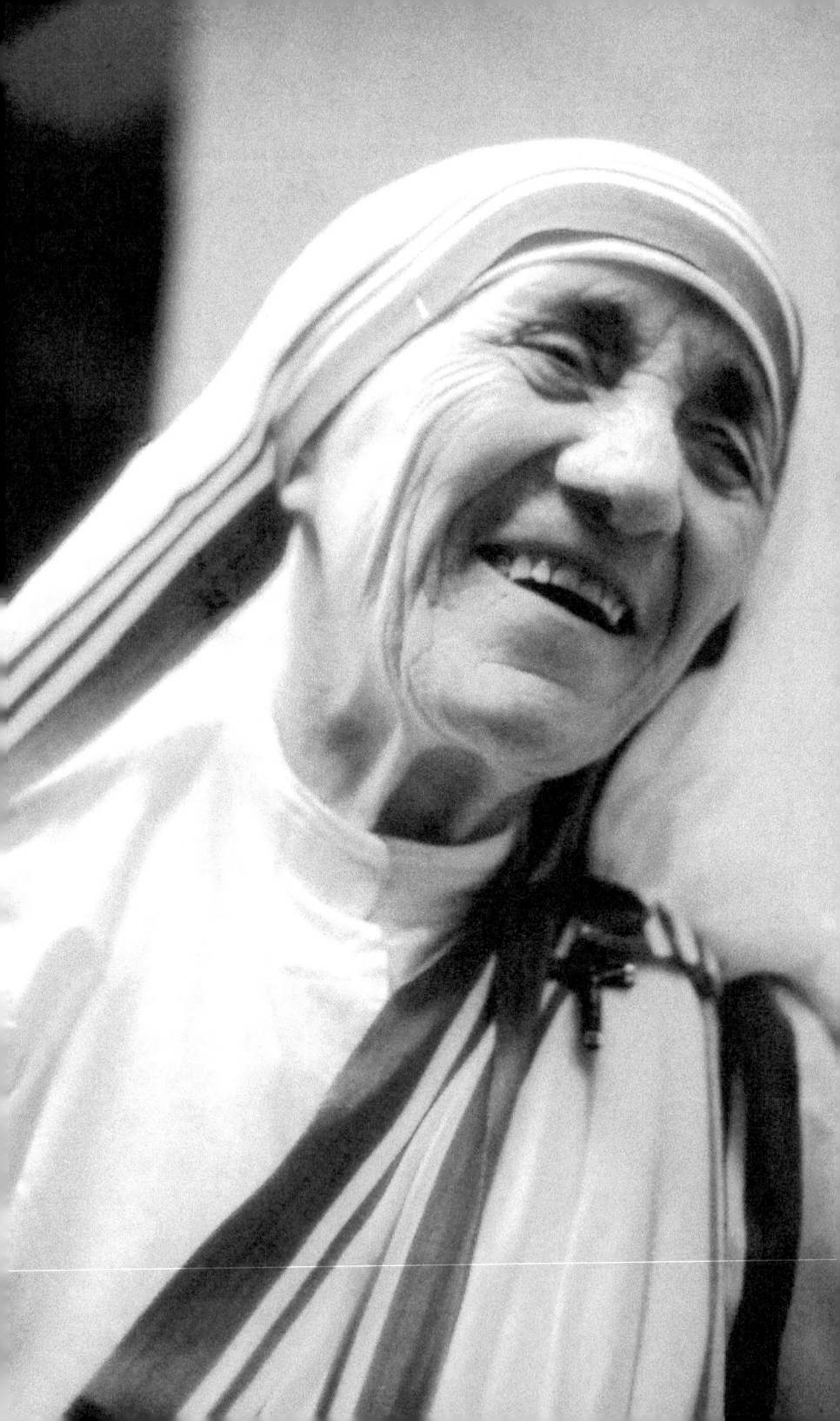

CHAPTER 1

You and Your Baby's
Value and Dignity

"How can there be too many children?
That is like saying there are too many flowers."

—St. Teresa of Calcutta

While preparing for my oldest son's fifteen-year well-child check, I was reminded of my seemingly endless nights of prayers to become pregnant. Growing up, I was that kid who wanted to be the neighborhood babysitter. Before I was ten, I remember wanting to hold the babies and help the moms in any way I could. Once I was married, and after more than seven years caring for other people's children as their registered nurse, I longed for a child of my own. My husband and I tried for over a year, and then just as we were seeking medical advice, I learned I was pregnant. The joy in my heart overflowed as a child of God grew in my womb.

We are all exquisitely created and one of a kind. God brings us into being on purpose. As my sweet boy's physical, emotional, and cognitive health grew, my spiritual health was being challenged from every angle. I knew I must respond to God's call for a closer relationship with Him in order to be the mom I wanted to be for our son.

> *"God created mankind in his image; in the image of God he created them; male and female he created them."*
>
> **—Genesis 1:27**

Our Lord loves us more than we can ever imagine. In fact, He created us in His image and likeness. He wants to be with us, walk with us, and dance with us during the joys of this life. He wants to rest with us when we are tired and encourage us when it is time to be courageous. He wants to hold us when we are at the end of our human journey. He asks us to care for ourselves as He is knitting our dear little ones in our wombs.

I think of Mother Mary when she learned that she was going to be pregnant with our Savior. Her first response was "How can this be . . ." (Luke 1:34). Maybe your response was the same! God calls us to surrender to Him and His will. Our heavenly Mother serves as the perfect example. Her next response to Gabriel was "May it be done to me according to your word" (Luke 1:38). Mary sought God and surrendered to His will. Next, she lovingly ran to a fellow daughter of God, her cousin Elizabeth. She joyfully exclaimed her excitement and then served Elizabeth, who was advanced in years and expecting John the Baptist!

Late in her pregnancy, Mary made the arduous journey to Bethlehem. We don't know what she had to endure as she rode on the donkey. Her fears, joys, and anticipations aren't described. All we know from the Bible is that after her son was born, she "kept all these things, reflecting on them in her heart" (Luke 2:19). The miraculous experience of our Savior born in such humble circumstances is locked inside her immaculate heart. Only a mother understands the experiences leading up to her child's birth and the bond that is unbreakable.

Mary teaches us that God meets us where we are and provides. He asks us to reflect on Him and His truth. He wants to transform us into the women He created us to be. To do this, we must say "yes" and nurture our whole beings. When a woman is pregnant, the Lord is growing a uniquely exceptional child in her womb. At the same time, He is yearning to grow a closer relationship with her.

Pregnancy

"You formed my innermost being; you knit me in my mother's womb. I praise you, because I am wonderfully made; wonderful are your works!"

—Psalm 139:13–14

Just as we are all uniquely created, each pregnancy experience is distinct. The classic symptom of nausea ruled the first sixteen weeks of my first pregnancy. I had plain Cheerios by my bed and snacked on them before I even lifted my head from the pillow upon awakening. Only recently can I enjoy lemon and ginger tea again! The second trimester was like a dream, for which I am extremely grateful. This quickly changed at thirty-six weeks, as I was in a fender bender and had to be hospitalized three times for intense contractions. At thirty-nine weeks, my water broke, and after thirty-two hours of labor and eight hours of pushing, Evan Walker was born at nine pounds, nine ounces. The nurse had to leave the delivery room to get larger diapers because the newborn size was not going to do the job!

My first child's personality was and continues to be what many professionals call "spirited." So, when my second husband, Keith, wanted us to get pregnant, I was not sure I was up for the task. Despite being thirty-eight, I agreed to lean in and trust God's plan. Within six months, I was ecstatic to tell my husband we were expecting.

My challenges with this pregnancy quickly became apparent. My diabetes went from controlled with diet and exercise to needing an insulin pump and continuous glucose monitoring. The next health challenge included anemia that impacted me enough to cause weakness, very low blood pressure, dizziness, and a couple fainting spells. As our baby grew, I experienced swelling in my legs and fluid around my heart. My blood pressure dropped whenever I stood up. Ultimately, I was put on bed rest for the last six weeks of the pregnancy. Throughout all of this, I was determined to keep being the mom I wanted to be for Evan, my nearly eight-year-old boy. Together we spent time reading, playing board games (backgammon was a favorite!), and watching movies.

As I reflect on those very challenging times, I realize the Lord was carefully knitting His children in my womb. He was weaving His love and His truth into their hearts, leaving a very special place only He can fill for them. The Lord was also transforming me throughout each pregnancy to become the mother I was called to be. Everyday choices became an opportunity to recognize my babies' value and dignity, practice self-care, and recognize the need for a sense of humor! In order to be healthy for their growing bodies, I was able to honor my children with my actions. My eating habits, ensuring I drank enough liquids, monitoring my blood pressure and blood sugar levels, and going to multiple doctor's appointments became a partnership with God to demonstrate my love. The way I could actively give God glory was to fulfill the demands of being a pregnant woman and recognize my baby's value and dignity. This meant nurturing my whole health.

Here are some practical tips:

- **Practice carving out time** to fill your mind with God's Word; let His love and peace support your growing spiritual health.

- **Attend** all required doctor's appointments.

- **Keep a journal** for any questions you have. At appointments, you can ask the doctor and write the answers for later reference.

- **If you have nausea,** be sure to talk with your provider about possible solutions. Sometimes little adjustments such as eating smaller, more frequent meals can be helpful. Ginger tea or ginger ale may be beneficial as well. For more severe nausea, your doctor may prescribe medication. Be careful with herbal supplements, though; many of them have unwanted side effects, so talk to your doctor or midwife if you plan to take any.

- **Stay hydrated,** as dehydration can cause premature contractions or lead to other health-related concerns.

- **Get your sleep,** even if in little naps! During pregnancy with my youngest son, I was so exhausted that I literally wanted to curl up underneath my desk at work and sleep! Consider going to the breastfeeding room and taking a ten-minute nap or having some moments of quiet time planned throughout the day.

- **Prevent constipation.** The saying "An apple a day, keeps the doctor away" was created for a reason! Fresh fruits and vegetables and whole grains keep the gut happy. Talk to your doctor early and often about constipation; it can be completely disruptive to your day!

- **Take a daily prenatal vitamin.** Buy what you can afford, and initially buy in the smallest quantity available. That way, if you cannot tolerate it, you can try a different vitamin. Don't take gummy prenatal vitamins as these are missing some of the essential nutrients you need to keep you and your baby healthy.

- **If you have anemia,** find a gentle iron supplement that is protein-bound; that tends to be easier on the stomach.

- **If you have diabetes,** know that your baby is at risk for heart conditions (also known as congenital heart disease). As a mom that required insulin for diabetes control and a former pediatric cardiology nurse, I urge all moms with diabetes to please see a specialist who can help you manage your blood sugar levels, eat foods high in protein, and follow your recommended carbohydrate load.

- **For ankle swelling,** wear knee-high compression stockings. These can make a huge difference. Discuss with your medical provider what type and level of compression the stockings should be.

- **Exercise during pregnancy** is important. Regular physical activity may help improve physical and mental health and may have positive benefits on labor and delivery. Since each pregnancy is different, speak with your obstetrician about what type of exercise would be best for your pregnancy.

- **Up to 90 percent of women get stretch marks** when pregnant. Following the above advice regarding hydration, nutrition, and exercise may help reduce the risk of stretch marks. Using moisturizing creams may also help reduce the chance of developing skin changes. Use whatever lotion you enjoy putting on your skin. While these prevention methods may help reduce the appearance of stretch marks, they aren't guaranteed to prevent them completely.

Reflect on God's truths and know that we are all His children. The child inside of your womb is God's child, and you are called to honor their dignity. By taking care of yourself, you are nurturing your baby and honoring your God-given value.

Delivery

Most pregnant women spend a great deal of time thinking about and planning their deliveries. Women speak with friends and family about the experiences they have had and form their own ideas about how they would prefer to deliver. Yet sometimes it's better to hand control over to God in these situations. As Isaiah 55:8 reminds us, God's thoughts are not our thoughts, and His ways are not ours. Give the reins to Him and let Him guide you during and after delivery.

NICOLE'S BIRTH STORY

Given the extensive labor and delivery process I went through with Evan, our obstetrician recommended a C-section for my second son. This was a fairly easy decision for me given that I later learned that the risk of hemorrhage and complications for the baby increases the longer labor continues. I was stubborn about the first delivery and insisted that if my vital signs and my son's fetal heart rate were normal, then I wanted a vaginal delivery. While I know that a vaginal delivery is ideal for mother and baby; sometimes circumstances do call for a C-section.

Keith and I decided to be open-minded, listen to the doctor, and pray about where we were guided for everyone's safety. The ultrasound showed that the amount of amniotic fluid was increasing and the baby was measuring as "very large." He was so large that I was even enrolled in a research study for a new ultrasound technique supposed to be more accurate in predicting the infant's weight!

Keith and I had great peace about the C-section, and we felt grateful for the gift of time to make the decision calmly. Baby Charles joined the world with the song "Come Holy Spirit" by Francesca Battistelli playing in the operating room. He was born weighing 10 pounds 5 ounces and was 22.4 inches long. The leaders of the ultrasound research later told me that he is an "outlier" in their data. I have to laugh as he continues to be a bit of a beautiful outlier!

Recovering from the C-section was similar to recovering from the prolonged vaginal delivery I had previously. I am old enough now to have heard a multitude of beautiful birth stories and also know a handful of heart-wrenching ones that ended tragically. I encourage everyone to read the facts from reputable resources and have open conversations with your trusted obstetrician or nurse midwife. If in doubt, seek a second opinion. And always seek the guidance of the Holy Spirit.

"For I know the plans I have for you, says the Lord, plans for welfare and not for evil, to give you a future and a hope."

—Jeremiah 29:11, RSVCE

KATHRYN'S BIRTH STORY

I was forty-one weeks pregnant with my third child and eager to deliver! I was admitted to the hospital in labor, and before long I was 7cm dilated. I assumed my delivery would be fast and easy, as it had been with my second child. After several hours of no change in status, my obstetrician decided to break my water.

Moments after my water broke, however, she realized that a very dangerous complication had occurred. My son's umbilical cord had "prolapsed," which means that it started to come down the birth canal before him. This emergency situation requires an immediate caesarean section. I started crying as multiple nurses entered the room. They urgently wheeled me into the operating room, where the last thing I remember was the obstetrician standing over me saying, "When can I start?"

When I woke up from the general anesthesia, my husband told me that our son was in stable condition but had to be taken to the neonatal intensive care unit to receive breathing support. My husband wasn't present for the delivery since I was under general anesthesia, and therefore, neither of us has a memory of the moment our son was born. His birth did not go at all how I expected, and this taught me some valuable lessons.

When things do not go as expected during delivery, a variety of emotions arise. Anxiety and fear or sadness and even anger can impact the first hours or days with your new baby. For those new mothers who experience complications, a prolonged hospitalization, or whose babies have to go to the neonatal intensive care unit, know that God sees you and is with you throughout those moments. Know that whatever you are journeying through, God has a plan for you, your baby and family.

Each Birth Story Is Sacred

Throughout this journey of pregnancy and childbirth, it is evident that God intertwines spiritual and physical aspects of health. Just as Mary's faith carried her through her extraordinary pregnancy, modern mothers can find strength in knowing that God is intimately present in every moment of their journey. We diligently attend to the practical aspects of maternal health through nourishing our bodies, seeking medical care, and preparing for birth. These efforts are more than just self-care. They are acts of worship, honoring both the Creator and the precious life He is forming within.

Yet perhaps the most profound lesson we can learn from both Mary's story and our own experiences is that God's perfect plan often unfolds in unexpected ways. When birth plans change or challenges arise, we can rest in the truth that every child's story is being written by the same loving Father who formed them in their mother's womb. This understanding brings dignity to every mother's experience, whether straightforward or complex, and reminds us that each birth story is sacred, each mother valuable, and each child fearfully and wonderfully made in His image.

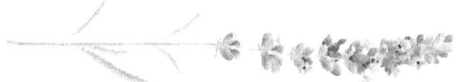

READ: *"For from him and through him and for him are all things. To him be glory forever."* (Romans 11:36)

MEDITATE: How is God asking you to show love to yourself and your growing child?

PRAY: Lord, reveal to me how I can embrace my changing body. Transform me into the mother my child needs me to be. Grant me the grace to embrace the demands of pregnancy and to wholly participate in growing the baby You have gifted me with! Amen.

LISTEN: "King of My Heart" by Bethel Music

RESOLVE:

1. Choose a small journal to write about your changing body and any questions for your doctor.
2. In your journal, write a Bible verse or a short prayer—or draw an image of encouragement to frequently reflect on throughout each day.

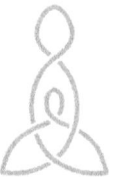

CHAPTER 2

Our Cornerstone and Light Source

"We must continually have before our eyes our model,
the exemplary life of Jesus Christ. We are called
to imitate this life."

—St. Louise de Marillac

A building's foundation or cornerstone serves to keep an entire building steady and prevent it from falling. Jesus as our cornerstone is often used as an analogy for living a life grounded in God's truth. Jesus also serves as our source of pure light and love, and with Him alone can we genuinely love ourselves and others.

St. Louise de Marillac, the patron saint of Christian social workers, is known for co-founding the Daughters of Charity, a community of sisters devoted to serving the most needy among us. Her work first began in 1633 with St. Vincent de Paul to meet the poorest and most abandoned in France.[6] In time, the ministry grew worldwide, and today it is a beacon of hope and charity.

6   "Saint Louise de Marillac," Catholic Online, accessed April 28, 2025, https://www.catholic.org/saints/saint.php?saint_id=196.

Louise was born in 1591 in France. She never knew her mother, who died when she was young. Her father was part of an affluent and influential French family, and though he loved Louise greatly, his new wife (Louise's stepmother) never truly accepted Louise as part of their family. Though Louise desired entrance into a convent, her initial application was rejected, and she entered into an arranged marriage. Prior to beginning the Daughters of Charity, St. Louise de Marillac was mother to a premature child with learning and growth disabilities.[7] Though she had a relatively compatible marriage, her husband developed an incurable illness after several years, and Louise devoted herself to caring for him. During the time she served her husband as his nurse, she suffered from depression and continued to think about the desire she had at a younger age to enter religious life. Several years after her husband passed away, in 1625 she met St. Vincent de Paul, and her life changed.

The saint practiced whole health for herself, her child, and her husband before embracing the call to serve those not related to her. She advocated for a strong spiritual health as the foundation upon which other health practices were based. Working alongside St. Vincent de Paul and subsequently other women, she ensured orphans received basic necessities such as food, shelter, and clothing. For the sick, she found placement in hospitals. For the poor, she offered job training and taught reading and writing. She fought for improved prison conditions. Interwoven in all her service was love, compassion, and kindness to meet the emotional needs of the people she encountered.

All of her actions, first for her immediate family and then for her community, were based on the truths of the Gospel. We are called

---

7   "Louise de Marillac and the World of Disability," DePaul University Digital Museum of Modern Art, May 8, 2023, https://blogs.depaul.edu/dmm/2023/05/08/louise-de-marillac-and-the-world-of-disability/.

to accept God's love and light, keep our eyes fixed on Him, and act according to His will. This starts at home as we nurture whole health for ourselves and our children.

> *"For you were once darkness, but now you are light in the Lord. Live as children of light, for light produces every kind of goodness and righteousness and truth."*
>
> **—Ephesians 5:8–9**

Jesus declares Himself "the light of the world," offering a path full of light for those who follow Him. When we align our lives with His teachings, His light dispels darkness and guides us toward truth, righteousness, and an abundant life. By wholeheartedly following Jesus, we become bearers of His light to the world around us. When we become mothers, this mission transforms into something even more beautiful. We are now called to shine His light not just to the world, but also to the new life He has entrusted to us. Through the gift of motherhood, we have the amazing opportunity to reflect His love and light to our children every single day.

By following Jesus, we embrace His love, mercy, and grace, allowing His light to penetrate every aspect of our being. As Scripture tells us, "The light shines in the darkness and the darkness has not overcome it" (John 1:5). Through this light, we discover the clarity, hope, and purpose that God intends for us. It leads us away from the shadows of falsehood, selfishness, and emptiness into a life filled with love, joy, and peace. As moms caring for our children, our words and actions can radiate the transformative love and power of His presence. He graces us with the ability to live faithfully and selflessly, bringing hope and love to our children and family. The more closely we align ourselves with Jesus, the more we reflect the glory of God to those we encounter.

When we open our hearts to God's creative power, we participate in His divine plan of bringing new life into the world. The vocation of motherhood is a sacred calling that reflects His unconditional love through our nurturing care and devotion to our children. As Scripture reminds us, "Her children rise up and call her blessed" (Proverbs 31:28).

Through motherhood, we unite our plan with God's vision, helping our children grow in His love while nurturing them with tenderness, compassion, and patience. This role shapes our spiritual journey and our children's character. God also calls us to honor our physical, emotional, cognitive, and spiritual health. This ever-evolving balancing act is challenging, yet it forms the foundation for optimal well-being for ourselves and our families.

Motherhood is celebrated as a profound expression of human value and dignity, a testament to the beauty of God's creation. Through the act of giving birth and raising children, we embody the divine image within us and impart it to our children. In this sacred role, we express unique qualities of femininity: compassion, tenderness, and selflessness. By embracing both our motherhood and our femininity, we embody a beautiful manifestation of the divine within the human experience. In motherhood, we catch a glimpse of the unconditional love and care that God bestows upon us as His children.

Nurturing Whole Health

The journey of giving birth and becoming a mom touches and reshapes every aspect of health, from the spiritual and physical to the cognitive and emotional. This book presents whole health for moms and babies grounded in the belief that God wants to guide and guard each of us. During the first year of life, all mothers have an opportunity to grow spiritually while their babies grow physically, cognitively, and emotionally.

Through love, we receive the grace to influence our child's character and values, molding them to be confident, courageous, and creative. We show this love through daily acts of service: feeding, soothing, diapering, clothing, and rocking. Each gentle response to our child's needs creates a healthy environment that nurtures each of us. These seemingly simple actions reflect the sacred nature of our vocation and manifest God's love in visible ways.

Fellow mamas in Christ, please hear this truth: Just as God tells us that our children have inherent dignity and value, recognize that the same applies to you as well. We moms serve as a reminder of our status as beloved children of God. We are a reflection of God's love and a reminder of our ongoing journey of growth and transformation as we strive to embody our divine calling and become the women God created us to be.

As we live this sacred calling of motherhood, our influence extends far beyond our homes. *Sacrificial love* and *self-giving* are not familiar or popular terms in today's culture. Society unceasingly teaches us to focus on our individual desires and goals. Now, more than ever, Catholic moms have an opportunity to have a profound and positive impact on society. Though sometimes our sphere of influence seems small, it truly does extend beyond our immediate family. Living as courageous mothers committed to selfless giving contributes to formation of a just and compassionate society. Caring actions rooted in love nurture a culture of respect, kindness, and joy. The power of daily choosing God's will ultimately fosters a society that embraces mercy, compassionate justice, and courageous creativity.

A mother's love, rooted in her deep sense of human dignity, promotes a culture of life and respect for all persons, from conception to natural death. Through her example and teachings, a mother instills in her children the values of compassion, mercy, and justice, helping to build a society that cherishes every human life. Through selfless love and nurturing care, we have an opportunity to reflect the image of God and shape the future of society. The choice is ours.

> *"The disciples rebuked them, but Jesus said, 'Let the children come to me, and do not prevent them; for the Kingdom of heaven belongs to such as these.'"*
>
> **—Matthew 19:14**

This world will present obstacles to prevent you and your child from seeking and going to Jesus. Remain steadfast. Just as a gardener tends to a garden to encourage the most beautiful and complete bloom, we must choose to daily tend to all aspects of whole health. We have an opportunity to encourage Jesus' light to shine brightly in ourselves and our children by nurturing whole health. Our love and caring actions reflect the authentic and unconditional love of God.

As children of God, we are constantly growing and evolving. Motherhood represents a transformative journey where we witness the growth and development of our children. Similarly, we are called to strive for spiritual growth and to more fully become the moms God has created us to be. The more His truth guides our thoughts and actions, the more we walk this journey of life with light, peace, and joy.

Promoting Your Baby's Whole Health Potential

Your baby's physical, spiritual, cognitive, and emotional health are interconnected aspects of overall well-being. Nurturing their spiritual health helps them develop a sense of purpose, their values, and a connection to something greater than themselves. It cultivates their moral compass and provides them with inner strength and resilience. Simultaneously, prioritizing their physical health ensures their bodies are strong, energized, and able to fully engage in life. Promoting cognitive and developmental health in children is also crucial for their future success and ability to thrive. Supporting children's emotional and social health creates the foundation for healthy relationships and resilient well-being. It encompasses nurturing their emotional intelligence, developing strong bonds, and equipping them with vital social skills. By nurturing our baby's whole health, we support our children in becoming well-rounded individuals who can navigate life's challenges, contribute positively to society, and experience a sense of holistic well-being. The following pages provide an initial overview of how you can promote the spiritual, physical, cognitive, and emotional health of your baby before diving deeper into various aspects of these topics in later chapters.

Spiritual Health

Fostering the spiritual well-being of children is a sacred responsibility that begins in the earliest moments of life. As parents, we have the privilege of planting seeds of God's mercy and love. The first steps of guiding our little ones into a deep and meaningful relationship with God begins very early in their lives. By creating an environment rich in faith, love, and devotion, we lay a foundation that will shape their character and influence their choices for years to come.

INFANCY: LAYING THE FIRST STONES

The spiritual journey can begin from the very first days of life. Simple yet intentional practices help nurture a child's innate connection to God:

- **Pray while rocking or feeding:** Speak to God out loud as you rock or feed your baby. Your words not only invite divine presence but also stimulate your child's developing mind. Studies show that the more words a baby hears, the stronger their cognitive growth.

- **Introduce Scripture early:** Reading a children's Bible to your baby creates familiarity with biblical language and stories. It establishes a rhythm of spiritual nourishment, even before comprehension begins.

- **Engage with faith-based toys:** Once your baby can grasp objects, provide soft, biblically themed toys. A plush Noah's Ark or a fabric book with Bible stories can serve as gentle, interactive introductions to faith.

- **Prioritize church attendance:** Attending church with an infant can be challenging, but the habit begins a routine that will become second nature as they grow. Even if much of the service is missed, the act of showing up honors God and establishes a family tradition of worship.

MODELING FAITH IN DAILY LIFE

Children are keen observers. Their earliest lessons in faith come not from formal instruction but from witnessing their parents live out Christian values.

- **Be a role model:** Let your child see you pray, read Scripture, and engage in acts of kindness. Modeling a life of faith teaches more than words ever could.

- **Show Christlike love:** Demonstrate patience, humility, and grace in daily interactions. How you respond to challenges and treat others shapes your child's understanding of Christian behavior.

PRAYING FOR AND WITH CHILDREN

One of the most powerful gifts a parent can offer is consistent prayer for their child's spiritual growth.

- **Create sacred rhythms of prayer:** Begin simple routines like praying before meals or at bedtime. These little moments plant seeds of connection with God that will grow with time. Don't underestimate the holiness of little prayers throughout the day—small whispers while preparing for bed or while singing a lullaby.

- **Worship as a family:** Interweave faith practices into the day by letting your home echo with worship. Humming hymns, playing Christian music, or reading Bible stories aloud create moments of truth and beauty of God's love. Oftentimes quick prayers, such as a Glory Be, can provide moments of family togetherness and centering.

- **Nurture wonder and truth:** From the very beginning, speak God's Word over your child. Use board books with Scripture, respond to their curious looks or pointing fingers, and pray out loud over their little lives. You're shaping their mind and their eternal soul.

Guiding a child on the path toward holiness is a sacred calling. By incorporating faith into everyday life through prayer, worship, biblical teaching, and church involvement, parents can nurture a lifelong relationship between their children and God. These small yet significant steps build a spiritual foundation that will carry them through every stage of life, firmly rooted in Christ's love.

Physical Health

WELL-CHILD VISITS THE FIRST TWELVE MONTHS— WHAT TO EXPECT

Combining physical, cognitive and emotional health with the central pillar of spiritual health fosters a whole health approach. Regular visits to a pediatrician or nurse practitioner help optimize physical health. During the first twelve months of a child's life, well-child visits are crucial for monitoring your baby's growth and development.

The American Academy of Pediatrics recommends a schedule of regular check-ups. Here is a summary of the well-child visit schedule:

- **Newborn:** Within the first week of birth, an initial visit is conducted to assess your baby's general health, perform necessary screenings, and address any concerns.

- **One month:** This visit focuses on your baby's feeding, growth, and development. Your healthcare provider addresses any concerns and provides guidance on sleep patterns and safety.

- **Two, four, and six months:** Your healthcare provider assesses your baby's developmental milestones and physical growth. Vaccinations are typically administered at these visits. Feeding and sleep patterns are topics of focus.

- **Nine months:** Your healthcare provider evaluates your baby's progress, development, and feeding habits. Concerns and questions are addressed and guidance on safety as your baby begins to explore their environment is discussed.

- **Twelve months:** This visit focuses on your baby's growth, development, and transitioning to whole milk and more solid foods. Vaccinations are administered, and your healthcare provider discusses future developmental milestones.

Depending on particular concerns or questions that you or your health care provider may have, more frequent visits may be required to closely follow the health of your infant.

Cognitive Health

Your baby's brain grows rapidly during the first three years of life. Encouraging brain cell connections in the early years lays the framework for intellectual development through school and the remainder of their lives. Wow! What a gift we moms have to positively impact our children in such a tremendous way! Here are a few initial tips (more will be discussed in Chapter 13):

- **Read books** out loud early and often.
- **Listen to music.** Research reveals music encourages brain synapse connections.
- **Talk and pray** with your baby. The more words and different sounds, the better.
- **Encourage their natural curiosity** by playing together, laughing, and smiling.

Emotional Health

Emotional health is the foundation for mental well-being. By promoting emotional awareness and regulation, children develop resilience, coping mechanisms, and self-confidence. They learn to recognize and express their emotions in healthy ways, which can help prevent the development of mental health issues later in life. Emotional health also contributes to a positive self-concept and healthy self-esteem. A positive self-image provides a solid foundation for future personal growth and achievement.

Here are some practical tips to promote emotional health:

- Holding, rocking, and talking to your baby encourages healthy attachment.
- Model empathy, compassion, and kindness in daily interactions. Infants as young as six months begin picking up on interactions and social cues.
- When your baby expresses their emotions, respond with encouragement, curiosity, and love.
- Consider teaching baby sign language to promote effective communication skills. Even learning basic signs such as *more, please, thank you,* and *hunger* help tremendously!
- Play with your baby early and often, such as during tummy time. You will be surprised how a short time together goes

a long way! Consider trying art, music, and physical exercise for different types of play.

- Begin to encourage self-soothing techniques at about three months of age.

Equip children, early and often, with the necessary tools to navigate life's challenges. The time spent is an investment in their long-term well-being and sets the foundation for a fulfilling and thriving future.

Be Committed to Whole Health

Remember, my sweet sisters in Christ, God's love for you and your child surpasses all understanding. God wants us to reflect His light. He wants us to reveal His divine qualities of nurturing, protection, and guidance that are characteristic of God's parental care. Commit to nurturing whole health—spiritual, physical, cognitive, and emotional—for you and your baby. Know God wants us to seek Him and to be near us while we walk the journey of motherhood. Turn to Him throughout your days and nights and He will show you how to be the mom you have been called to be.

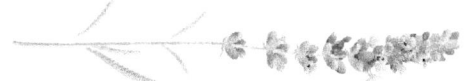

READ: *"Remember. . . that you must take great care to help them to know and love our Lord."* (St. Louise de Marillac[8])

MEDITATE: Considering the four pillars of whole health—spiritual, physical, cognitive, and emotional—imagine what God wants for you and your baby.

PRAY: Dear heavenly Father, open the eyes of my heart. Help me to walk in your light as your child. Show me how to teach my child to do the same. Amen.

LISTEN: "You Say" by Lauren Daigle

RESOLVE:

1. Choose a child's book about faith to read to your baby daily. Bible stories, saints, God's love are a few examples.
2. Print a holy image or Bible verse that reminds you of God's love and place it in a prominent location in your home.

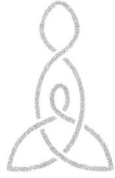

---

8   St. Louise de Marillac, *Spiritual Writings*, L. 548, p. 573.

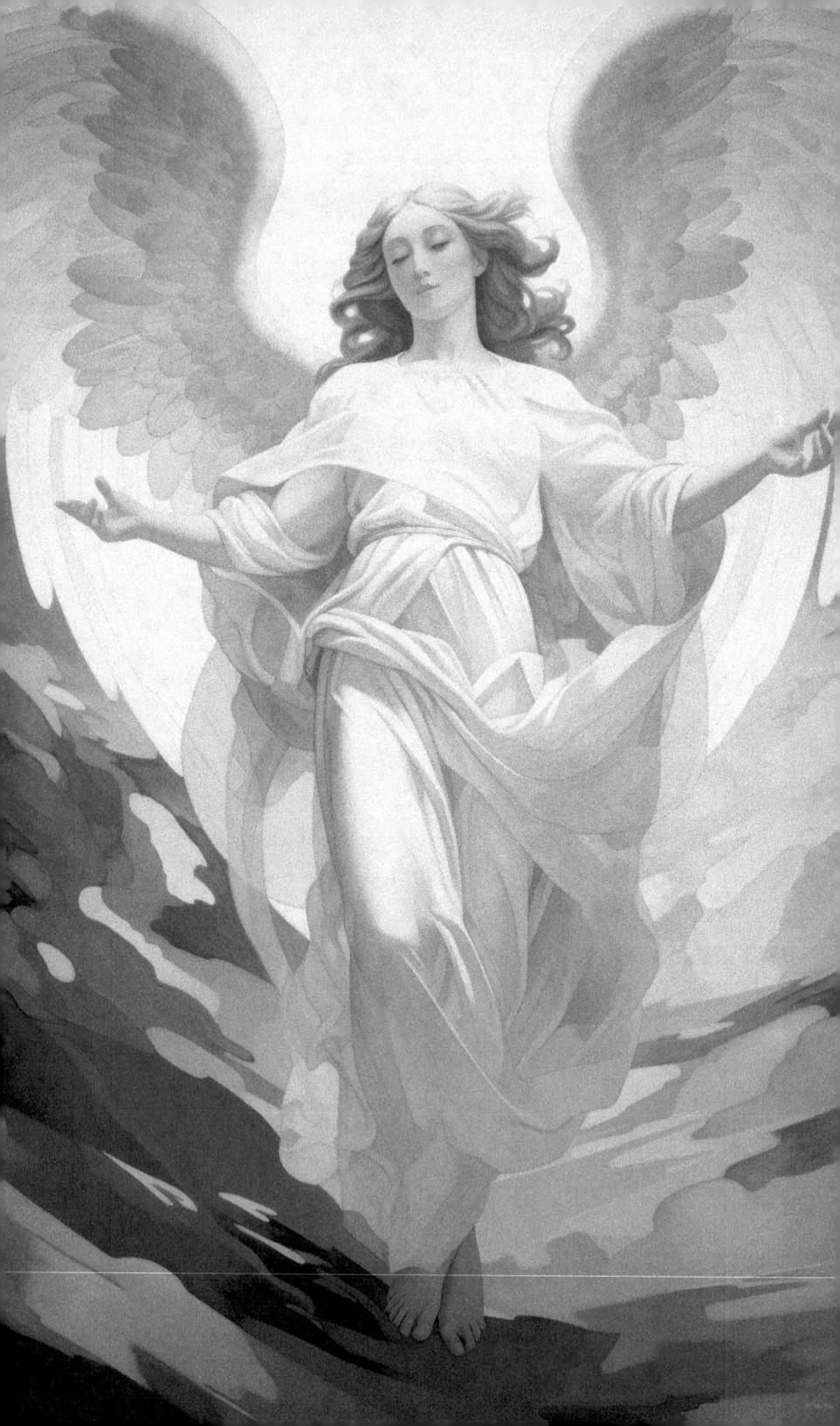

CHAPTER 3

Unconditional Love
and Constant Care

Both of my boys were born with only the slightest bit of hair. I fondly remember feeling their soft fuzzy heads against my cheek as I held them close. As I rocked them, I would pray they would calm down and doze off. As their cries became sighs and their bodies became less tense, feelings of relief would comfort me. The best feeling in the world is holding a baby as they begin to doze off to sweet sleep. Their complete trust becomes palpable in the way they let go and rest. I marvel knowing this is how God wants us to be with Him.

"Are not two sparrows sold for a small coin? Yet not one of them falls to the ground without your Father's knowledge. Even all the hairs of your head are counted."

—Matthew 10:29–30

Knowing and accepting God's love is central to understanding who He is and His relationship with each of us. God's love is selfless, unwavering, and boundless. God's love is freely given because it is rooted in His infinite mercy and compassion. We know that His love is unconditional because it is independent of what we have done or failed to do. Because we live in a fallen world, humanity finds this perfect love almost impossible to grasp. Despite our flaws and failures, He constantly reaches out to embrace with welcoming arms and heal all those who seek His love. God's love is a transformative force that nurtures spiritual growth. A personal and intimate relationship with Him is how we grow and flourish in His love.

We are called by name to have faith in His vast love by grasping His hand and saying, "Yes, Lord, I accept your love." God's unconditional love is exemplified in the life and sacrifice of Jesus Christ, who is the incarnation of God's love. God sent Jesus as a divine gift and promise of life everlasting with Him. Forgiveness and redemption are ours as his daughters. Jesus' teachings emphasize forgiveness, compassion, and the call to love one another as He loved us.

While God's care for us is always present to guide us and protect us, He knows our hearts and minds long to know that He sees us and cares about us. One of these ways is His gift to us of our own guardian angel specially designed to care for and watch over us.

> *"For He will command His angels concerning you*
> *to guard you in all your ways."*
>
> **—Psalm 91:11**

Jesus received loving care from angels when He walked among us. Matthew 4:11 tells us that angels attended to Him and encouraged Him as He obeyed His Father's will. In Hebrews 1:14, angels are mentioned as spiritual creatures sent by God to serve and minister to us. As we care for our children, our guardian angel is with us. Our children are also granted their own guardian angels to watch over them.

As mothers, we are graced with the ability to radiate God's love. God's unconditional love for all is mirrored in our motherly love for our children. We have a unique ability to provide nurturing care, guidance, and protection for our children. We have the opportunity to create a secure and loving environment for them to grow into the person God created them to be.

Our watchful and loving presence is precious because it offers a sense of comfort and reassurance to our children. With God's help, we create a strong foundation for our child's emotional and psychological development. We play a vital role in shaping our children's lives. Foundational to a healthy environment for optimal growth is prevention of illnesses and injury. Infants are completely dependent on us and rely on our unconditional love for them to nurture their growth and protect them from harm.

I am often asked, "What can I do to keep my baby from getting sick?" As mothers, we want to prevent the discomfort and complications associated with an illness or injury. This is a beautiful and loving desire mothers have for their children. While we know we all get sick at some point in time, we can practice ways to prevent illness and to decrease the severity and length of an illness. Injury prevention must be a high priority as the effects of illness can be fatal or have a long-lasting impact on health and wellness.

I often have to remind myself to go back to the basics. My boys now know my mantra well: "We eat, we sleep, and we pray." Life is full of distractions and demands. However, our minds, souls, and bodies were created in the image of God. He designed us intentionally. When we honor basic truths and listen to essential needs, we lay a strong foundation for thriving as He intends. Healthy eating, restful sleep, and intentional prayer time provide a strong foundation to build upon for illness and injury prevention.

Illness Prevention

Maintaining a clean environment, regular hand washing, and avoiding contact with those who have contagious conditions are excellent practices to help prevent illnesses. Here are four tips for preventing illnesses:

1. Attending regularly scheduled well-child visits is paramount to ensure your child is growing and developing in a way that can optimize their health and wellness. Well visits allow healthcare providers to assess how a child is growing and developing. Additionally, at these visits providers can identify illness or disease early. In fact, regular attendance at well-child visits has been linked to fewer hospitalizations and emergency room visits.[9] Well-child visits also offer counseling on ways to develop healthy habits for your infant and prepare you to know what to expect as your infant grows.

2. "Thank you for asking, but we prefer that our baby is not held at this time." It's okay to say no if someone asks to hold your baby! As a new mom, I thought there was an unwritten law that if someone asked to touch or hold my baby, I had to let them. Not true! If a well-meaning individual reaches into the car seat or bassinet to touch your baby's angelic cheeks, you have permission to say, "Please use the hand sanitizer first" or "We are protective and prefer our baby's face is not touched." Be ready to speak up so that when the time comes to defend your little one, you are ready! Be sure to have hand sanitizer strapped to your car seat or stroller if you do say yes.

3. Breast milk contains antibodies and essential nutrients that help strengthen the infant's immune system and may reduce the risk of various infections and illnesses. Some of the benefits

---

9   E.R. Wolf, J. O'Neil, J. Pecsok, R.S. Etz, D.J. Opel, R. Wasserman, and A.H. Krist, "Caregiver and Clinician Perspectives on Missed Well-Child Visits"," Annals of Family Medicine 18, no. 1 (January 2020): 30–34.

include decreased ear infections and respiratory illnesses such as pneumonia. Sudden Infant Death Syndrome prevalence is also lower in breastfed infants. The American Academy of Pediatrics recommends exclusive breastfeeding for the first six months of life. We recognize that breastfeeding can have challenges and may not be possible for every mother. Breastfeeding and formula will be discussed in further detail in Chapter 5.

4. Vaccinations are among the most powerful defenses we have to shield our children from infectious diseases and their potentially severe complications. A 2024 published report concluded that for children born between 1994 and 2023, routine childhood vaccinations will have prevented an estimated 508 million cases of illness, 32 million hospitalizations, and 1,129,000 deaths. These benefits result in direct savings of $540 billion and societal savings of $2.7 trillion.[10]

Vaccines approved by the Food and Drug Administration (FDA) undergo rigorous safety and effectiveness evaluation before being recommended for use. Medical and public health experts carefully review the evidence supporting each vaccine's safety and efficacy. Scientific consensus strongly supports following established immunization schedules for infants and children. In the first two years of life your child's immune defenses are most vulnerable. Therefore, following the established immunization schedule for preventable diseases is considered essential for protecting your child's health.[11] All of the recommended vaccines are given to prevent illness, costly hospitalizations, long-term morbidity, loss of work, and unnecessary loss of precious life.

10   F. Zhou, T.C. Jatlaoui, A.J. Leidner, et al. "Health and Economic Benefits of Routine Childhood Immunizations in the Era of the Vaccines for Children Program—United States, 1994–2023," MMWR Morbidity and Mortality Weekly Report 73 (2024): 682–685.

11   K.H. Nguyen, A. Srivastav, M.C. Lindley, A. Fisher, D. Kim, S.M. Greby, J. Lee, and J.A. Singleton, "Parental Vaccine Hesitancy and Association With Childhood Diphtheria, Tetanus Toxoid, and Acellular Pertussis; Measles, Mumps, and Rubella; Rotavirus; and Combined 7-Series Vaccination," American Journal of Preventive Medicine 62, no. 3 (March 2022): 367–376.

Due to the success of immunizations, many young families have thankfully never personally witnessed pertussis, measles, vaccine-preventable meningitis, or other diseases prevented by immunization. Unfortunately, when immunization rates drop, breakthrough cases or clusters of disease can occur, sometimes with serious results. It is particularly heartbreaking to care for an infant in the intensive care unit struggling to breathe due to pertussis, or to monitor a young child who is unresponsive with pneumococcal meningitis, knowing these cases may have been prevented with proper vaccination.

We want to highlight three common vaccine preventable diseases which we have had personal experience with in the hospital setting. We use these as examples to illustrate why vaccines are so vital to our health. We urge you to discuss these vaccines and all the recommended vaccines with your pediatric provider.

Pertussis, also known as whooping cough, is a bacterial infection that causes uncontrollable coughing. Though most adults will recover, infants and young children are most severely affected. In infants, the coughing fits can result in apnea (where babies stop breathing and turn blue due to lack of oxygen). Before the vaccine was developed, pertussis was one of the leading causes of death in infants. Pertussis caused between 115,000 to 270,000 cases each year and 5,000 to 10,000 deaths annually prior to vaccine availability.[12] The vaccine protects against pertussis, diphtheria, and tetanus, building a fortress of immunity for your little one.

Haemophilus influenzae type b (Hib) is a bacteria that causes ailments ranging from ear infections and pneumonia to life-threatening meningitis (a severe infection of the membrane that protects the

---

12   L. Merdrignac, F. Aït El Belghiti, E. Pandolfi, et al, "Effectiveness of One and Two Doses of Acellular Pertussis Vaccines Against Laboratory-Confirmed Pertussis Requiring Hospitalisation in Infants: Results of the PERTINENT Sentinel Surveillance System in Six EU/EEA Countries, December 2015–December 2019," *Vaccine* 42, no. 9 (April 2024): 2370–2379.

brain and spinal cord) and epiglottitis (a devastating infection which can block the windpipe, causing suffocation). In the United States, about twenty-thousand children under the age of five suffered from serious Hib infections annually and one thousand unfortunately died from the disease before the vaccine was available.[13] Among those who survived serious Hib infections, long term complications of the disease were common, including chronic seizures and hearing loss. With the introduction of the vaccine, the number of cases of invasive Hib have decreased by 99 percent.[14]

A third illness we want to focus attention on is rotavirus. This virus was a common cause of severe diarrhea. Before the introduction of the rotavirus vaccine, severe dehydration led to hospitalizations and even death. With the vaccine's integration into the immunization schedule, there has been a profound decrease in both the incidence and severity of rotavirus infections. The immunization effort has prevented an estimated 460,000 cases, 118,000 hospitalizations and 27 unnecessary deaths annually.[15]

While these specific examples highlight just a few of the recommended vaccines, all vaccines are given to prevent illness and protect the health and well-being of communities.

As with many medical breakthroughs, controversy and differing opinions exist. Everything we introduce into our bodies has the potential to cause side effects. Most vaccines may only cause very mild side effects but, extremely rarely, some vaccines may cause more serious adverse events. It is important to understand, however,

---

13   "Haemophilus Influenzae," Cleveland Clinic, accessed March 7, 2025. https://my.clevelandclinic.org/
      health/diseases/23106-haemophilus-influenzae.

14   "Haemophilus Influenzae Disease Surveillance," Centers for Disease Control and Prevention,
      accessed March 7, 2025, https://www.cdc.gov/hi-disease/php/surveillance/index.html.

15   A.T. Newall, R.N. Leong, J.F. Reyes, et al, "Rotavirus Vaccination Likely to Be Cost Saving to Society in
      the United States," Clinical Infectious Diseases 73, no. 8 (October 20, 2021): 1424–1430.

that vaccines have been studied extensively and *the benefits of vaccination clearly outweigh the risks*. Dozens of well-performed studies have shown that vaccines do not cause autism, asthma, diabetes, allergies, or brain damage. Infants are not too young to receive vaccines, and immunization does not suppress the immune system.[16]

Unfortunately, sometimes the ramifications of misinformation regarding vaccines can result in serious complications. Immunization rates for measles virus have been slowly dropping in many areas of the country, leading to the resurgence of a disease that was declared eliminated in the United States in 2000 by the CDC and World Health Organization.[17] Measles outbreaks in 2025 in Texas and New Mexico demonstrate how quickly this highly contagious virus can spread when community immunity falters. Before the measles vaccine was introduced in 1963, nearly every child contracted measles, resulting in approximately four hundred to five hundred deaths and thousands of hospitalizations annually in the United States alone. A single piece of discredited research (later retracted by the medical journal that published it) sparked widespread fear about the MMR vaccine, despite overwhelming scientific evidence confirming its safety. This illustrates how vulnerable public health can be to misinformation, especially when it comes to protecting our most defenseless populations. As both mothers and pediatric providers, we ask you to consider that choosing vaccination is not just about protecting your child, but about safeguarding all children in your community, including those too young to be vaccinated or with severe medical conditions that prevent immunization.

It is also important to discuss the Catholic position on vaccination. The Church supports vaccination as a socially responsible act to

---

16   "Vaccine Education Center," Children's Hospital of Philadelphia, accessed March 1, 2025, https://www.chop.edu/vaccine-education-center.

17   "Measles Data & Research," Centers for Disease Control and Prevention, accessed March 7, 2025, https://www.cdc.gov/measles/data-research/index.html.

protect individual and community health. While acknowledging moral concerns about vaccine development, particularly regarding cell lines derived from historical fetal tissue, the Church has clarified that receiving vaccines is morally acceptable, especially when no alternative vaccines are available. The Vatican has emphasized that receiving vaccines can be an act of charity, particularly when they help keep vulnerable populations safe. Pope Francis and other Catholic leaders have been clear that vaccination represents a practical way of showing concern for others and it aligns with the Catholic moral teaching of protecting human life.[18]

The statistics discussed above highlight the transformative benefits of vaccines. By keeping to the recommended vaccine schedule, you are not only ensuring your child's health but also contributing to the containment of these diseases, thus protecting the health of the community at large and that of future generations. We pray the information presented above strengthens your confidence in choosing vaccination to protect your infant and others.

Injury Prevention

Unintentional injury is a leading cause of death and disability for infants and children.

When practicing in a small town pediatric clinic, I was on call two or three nights a week. Unfortunately, many middle of the night calls were for concerns about injuries after a baby fell off a diaper-changing station, bed, swing, or other infant product. The incidents were always upsetting, scary, and unexpected. Some resulted in emergency room visits, and a few required hospitalization due to traumatic brain injuries. No parent wants to live through this scene.

---

18   "FAQ on the Use of Vaccines," National Catholic Bioethics Center, accessed March 1, 2025, https://www.ncbcenter.org/resources-and-statements-cms/faq-on-the-use-of-vaccines.

Accidents such as falls, drowning, accidental poisoning, and motor vehicle crashes occur every day in the United States and can have devastating consequences. Infants are particularly vulnerable due to their curiosity, limited understanding of danger, and developing motor skills. Parents need to be equipped with practical strategies to prevent unnecessary pain and suffering.

- **Car seats:** Always use a car seat when transporting your infant in a vehicle. Ensure the car seat is rear-facing until your child reaches the age of two. Be sure to check the specific height and weight limits recommended by the car seat manufacturer and ask your pediatrician if you have specific questions. The car seat should be properly installed according to the manufacturer's instructions and the vehicle's owner's manual. The harness straps should fit snugly, with the chest clip at armpit level. Do not place infants in a car seat with bulky clothing, blankets, snowsuits, or jackets under the straps. Local fire departments often offer free checks to make sure the car seat is properly installed.

- **Infant swings, bouncy chairs, and similar products:** Beginning with the first time you put your baby in the device, strap them in! This practice will ensure that the day your baby can wiggle out, they are safely secured. Build your muscle memory by practicing fastening the strap every time. Follow the manufacturer's guidelines for weight and age, and never leave your infant unattended in the swing.

- **Proper holding:** Your sweet little one has very immature neck muscles and needs your help supporting their head and neck. This will prevent any injury and give them a sure sense of security.

- **Risk of rolling:** Infants can roll over unexpectedly, so never leave them unattended on high surfaces like beds, changing tables, or sofas. The first roll can happen at any time and always when least expected.

- **Childproofing the home:** Before our youngest could crawl, my husband and I got on our hands and knees and went around the house to observe what we could see and reach. We were amazed at all the potentially hazardous items at ground level! Each parent has a threshold for baby proofing, and you need to feel comfortable with the practicalities and cost. Essentials include covering electrical outlets, securing cords, anchoring heavy furniture to the wall to prevent tipping, and keeping small objects that may cause choking out of reach. Install safety gates to prevent falls down stairs and use door locks to keep children away from dangerous areas. Store medicines, cleaning supplies, and other toxic materials in locked cabinets or out of reach. Use child safety locks on cabinets and ensure that any potentially poisonous plants are removed from the areas where your child can reach them. Keep the number for the poison control center handy in case of accidental ingestion.

- **Water safety:** One day, while in the bathroom with Charlie, I found myself distracted by my phone. Thankfully, nothing happened, but I realized I needed to be more focused on my son's safety. From that day on, the bathroom became a "no phone zone." Infants can drown in only two inches of water, so always keep a hand on your infant while in the bath, and drain the bath immediately after use. Consider taking baby swim classes together—this provides amazing fun and teaches practical measures for your baby to learn how to float and get out of a pool.

- **Product and toy recalls:** Unfortunately, not all infant products readily available in stores and online are actually safe.

Recalls indicate that a product has been found to compromise safety, potentially leading to injury or even death. Design flaws, manufacturing defects, or the use of harmful materials (such as lead) can lead to future recalls. Stay informed by getting notifications from government bodies or safety watchdog organizations. You can also proactively register products with manufacturers for direct notification.

- **Sun and heat exposure:** Protect infants by keeping them in the shade when possible and use sun hats and protective clothing. Use sunscreen sparingly for an infant under six months of age when you cannot avoid sun exposure. Over the age of six months, apply sunscreen liberally and often. Never leave an infant in a parked car, as the temperature inside a vehicle can rise quickly and lead to heatstroke.

- **Choking and suffocation prevention:** Keep small items out of infants' reach to prevent choking. It's surprising what infants and toddlers might try to put in their mouths. Toys should be evaluated carefully to ensure they do not have removable or easily breakable parts that may pose a choking hazard. Floors and low surfaces should be monitored regularly to ensure they are free from items that might pose a choking risk. Avoid giving infants foods that might become choking hazards (such as grapes and peanuts).

Safe Sleeping Habits

I think we can all agree that sleep is necessary for everyone to be at their best! Sleeping is one of the three essential building blocks of health. Safe sleep education is a passion of mine. Early in my nursing career, I learned about the potential deleterious effects of co-sleeping, and I believe all parents should be aware of this. This following story is sobering, and I share it out of love for you and your baby.

As a young ER nurse, I comforted a mom who inadvertently rolled over on her infant as she was sleeping. The paramedics brought her into the emergency room still holding her baby. She was crying and unable to accept the reality that her baby was no longer breathing. This was an awful experience that no mother should have to endure. Later in my career, I supported nurse colleagues who worked in the pediatric intensive care unit as they lamented over caring for infants now dependent on ventilators to breathe due to suffocation while sleeping. These experiences led me to try to educate as many parents as possible on proper safe sleep techniques.

I know there is no better feeling than holding a sleeping infant and listening to them breathe sweetly. But once you become at all sleepy yourself, please put your baby down into a safe sleeping position and environment. Sudden Infant Death Syndrome (SIDS) and other sleep-related deaths remain a significant concern, making it imperative for mothers to prioritize safe sleep practices. The American Academy of Pediatrics advises against bed-sharing. Instead, placing the crib or bassinet in the same room as the parents can provide the benefits of close proximity while maintaining a separate sleep surface for the infant.

Placing your infant on their back to sleep is the best position for an unobstructed airway and healthy breathing. A safe environment includes a firm and flat mattress with a fitted sheet. Remove all soft bedding, pillows, stuffed animals, and bumper pads from the crib. Do not use a nursing pillow or any other products marketed as a sleep aid in the crib or sleeping environment. A bassinet, portable crib, or other flat surface with protective barrier walls or rails is best.

Mothers play a critical role in establishing safe sleep habits for their children. By following recommended practices, you can protect your children from sleep-related incidents and promote healthy sleep patterns from the earliest stages of life.

Safe Crying

Despite meeting all of an infant's needs such as diaper changing, feeding, and soothing, crying can persist. This is not because you have failed in some way. Commonly, infants go through a unique developmental time period when they can cry significantly for no apparent reason. Some experts refer to this as the "period of PURPLE crying," while others may use the older term *colic*. This challenging phase may typically begin at two to three weeks of age and last until the baby is three to four months old.[19] Becoming familiar with "PURPLE crying" helps caregivers anticipate and accept this normal developmental stage.

The acronym "PURPLE" outlines the distinctive aspects of this crying phase:

- **P**eak of crying: An increase in crying, peaking at around the second month and diminishing in the subsequent months.

- **U**nexpected: The onset of crying may seem sudden and without obvious cause.

- **R**esists soothing: The baby might continue to cry despite all attempts to calm them.

- **P**ain-like face: Infants may appear to be in pain, even when they are not.

- **L**ong-lasting: Crying bouts can stretch for several hours.

- **E**vening: The late afternoon and evening may bring more intense crying episodes.[20]

Even though this phase is common in infants, the intensity and persistence of the crying can be distressing. Now is the time to

---

19   C.N. Grier, L.A. Thompson, "What Parents Should Know About Crying in Infants," *JAMA Pediatrics* 178, no. 12 (December 1, 2024): 1379.

20   "PURPLE Crying," National Center on Shaken Baby Syndrome, accessed April 11, 2025, https:// dontshake.org/purple-crying.

recognize and practice your coping skills. There are several commonly recommended soothing techniques that may help if your baby is crying. Try wrapping your infant securely in a swaddle to recreate womb-like security or introducing soothing background sounds such as white noise or rhythmic heartbeat recordings. Many babies respond well to gentle motion through rocking or carrier-wearing, while others may calm with non-nutritive sucking on a pacifier or clean finger. Gentle massage can also help, though always stay attentive to your baby's reactions.[21]

For potential gas discomfort, try positioning strategies like cradling your baby face down along your forearm while supporting their head, or gently moving their legs in bicycle motions when they're on their back. While these approaches frequently help calm distressed infants, remember that some crying episodes naturally need to run their course.[22] During these challenging moments, recognize that your loving presence matters even when immediate soothing isn't possible.

If you are concerned that these crying episodes may be something more serious, contact your pediatric provider right away. This is especially important if you notice decreased feedings, fever, vomiting, or decreased activity level. Also watch for changes in alertness, areas of swelling or redness, or any other unusual changes in your baby's behavior or appearance.[23]

During the "period of "PURPLE crying," it is also essential to recognize when you are becoming overwhelmed. You may experience feelings of frustration, impatience, and helplessness. Physical signs of stress might include muscle tension and headaches, while emotional

---

21   "PURPLE Crying: What It Is and How to Cope," What to Expect, accessed April 11, 2025, https://www. whattoexpect.com/first-year/care/purple-crying#tips.

22   "PURPLE Crying," What to Expect.

23   "PURPLE Crying," Cleveland Clinic, last reviewed December 22, 2023, https://my.clevelandclinic.org/ health/articles/purple-crying.

indicators may include feelings of sadness, anxiety, desperation, or having doubts about your ability to manage the situation. These feelings can be a common part of the parenting journey.

Professionals advise that when overwhelmed, it is not only okay but necessary to place the baby in a safe environment and take a moment for yourself. Stepping out of the room allows you to engage in self-care, regain composure, and return to your infant calmer and more equipped to provide comfort.

During a self-imposed break, ask for God's grace and peace. Practicing deep breathing, calling a friend or family member, praying, or jogging in place are some examples that can help calm you. These moments of respite are crucial and can prevent the buildup of stress, ensuring that both baby and caregiver remain safe. Talking to others who understand can be a lifeline! Healthcare professionals can also serve to offer guidance and confirm that such experiences are common and manageable.

In your most vulnerable moments, remember that *it is imperative never to shake a baby*. If you ever feel you are on the brink of causing harm, it is critical to seek help immediately. "PURPLE crying" is challenging, but it never justifies harming an infant. It is a stage that will pass, and with the right support and knowledge, it can be navigated successfully. Remember, reaching out for support during this time is not a sign of weakness—it's a proactive step in ensuring the best care for both you and your infant. This phase shall pass, leaving behind a deeper understanding of infant care and an even stronger bond between you and your baby.

Safe Play

Encouraging safe play at an early age is crucial for infants' physical well-being and overall development. First, it is essential to create a safe play space. This includes ensuring that the area is free from hazards such as sharp objects, choking hazards, or dangerous equipment. Regularly inspecting play areas, both indoors and outdoors, can help identify and address potential safety concerns.

Supervision is key to ensuring safe play. Adults should actively watch children during playtime, particularly when they are engaged in activities that may involve risks. Being present allows caregivers to intervene if necessary and guide children in making safe choices.

Learning basic life support, which includes CPR and the Heimlich maneuver, builds confidence and provides essential skills that could help save lives. Parents have shared with me that knowing these skills made them feel more confident when enjoying outings with friends and family or being at home by themselves with their babies. Having the knowledge and skills to protect your infant and respond in emergencies brings peace of mind when it matters most.

Guarding and Protecting
Our Little Ones

"O give thanks to the Lord, for he is good;
for his steadfast love endures forever!"

—1 Chronicles 16:34

Parental love offers us a glimpse into the infinite, unconditional love God has for each of us. Just as God walks with us through all of our triumphs and struggles, we lead our own children through the joys and challenges of daily life. When we protect and nurture our children by following safe sleep practices, keeping them up to date on vaccinations, or taking steps to prevent illness or injuries, we work alongside the guardian angels God has gifted us.

For four years, I had the privilege of taking care of infants with congenital heart defects. One of the best parts of a nursing shift was when I could console a crying infant whose parents were not present for a multitude of reasons. Not a day went by that I didn't hold a baby at some point. During these moments while holding God's precious children, I witnessed infants being guarded and ministered to by their guardian angels.

As we care for our children, remember that each action to keep them healthy and safe is a reflection of God's love for us. He has blessed us with both medical knowledge and guardian angels to help guide our way. Trust in His presence as you navigate motherhood; you are never alone on this path.

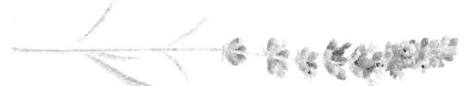

READ: The Catechism of the Catholic Church proclaims that *"from infancy to death human life is surrounded by their [angels'] watchful care and intercession. Beside each believer stands an angel as protector and shepherd leading him to life. Already here on earth the Christian life shares by faith in the blessed company of angels and men united in God"* (CCC, 336)

MEDITATE: Envision how God loves you so much that he gave you a guardian angel.

PRAY: Angel of God, my guardian dear, to whom God's love commits me here, ever this day be at my side, to light and guard, to rule and guide. Amen.

LISTEN: "Angel by Your Side" by Francesca Battistelli

RESOLVE:

1. Memorize the Guardian Angel prayer and say it daily with your baby.
2. What is one action that you can take to protect your baby from illness or injury?

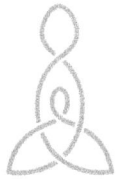

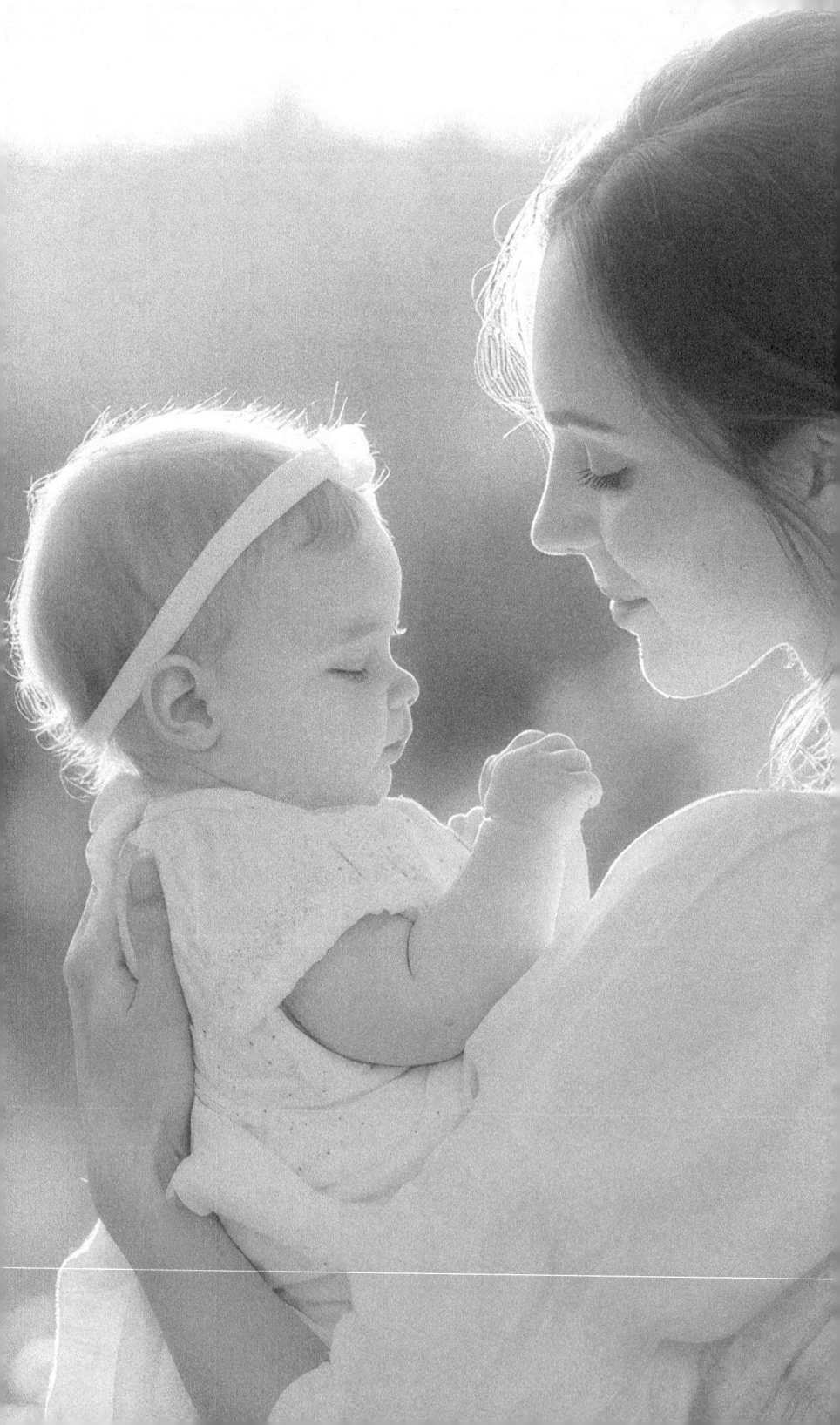

CHAPTER 4

Breaths of Life

"Then the LORD God formed the man out of the dust
of the ground and blew into his nostrils the breath of life,
and the man became a living being."

—Genesis 2:7

As a mom, I often find myself holding my breath! Joy, caution, anticipation, love, curiosity, and compassion are just a few of the emotions that overwhelm my heart. Becoming a mother introduced me to a spectrum of emotions, ranging from deep fear to overwhelming joy. One vivid memory stands out among them all— the moment I first saw my newborn. There, in the delivery room, the silence was broken by the sound of a nurse gently tapping the tiny feet of my baby. This simple act was to encourage my newborn to draw in a much-needed breath. The sight of his purple-tinged skin is etched in my memory, a visual testament to the tension that filled the room. I found myself unintentionally holding my own breath. The moment his lungs filled with air and he let out his first cry, a sound so profoundly moving, it imprinted on my heart as the most beautiful melody.

My professional journey as a nurse has been punctuated by numerous moments where the presence or absence of breath played a central role. Countless times, I've found myself in critical situations where a child's breath was labored or halted, and we, as a medical team, stepped in to become their breath, their lifeline. The weight of these moments is heavy, and often, I would catch myself holding my breath in solidarity with the struggling child. Every time we witnessed the rise of a chest or heard the steady beep of a monitor signaling stabilized vital signs, it was as if we all exhaled a collective sigh of relief, a momentary respite in the midst of chaos.

Now, as I've transitioned to the role of an educator, instructing the next generation of nurses, I emphasize the fundamental principle of patient care: the ABCs: Airway, Breathing, and Circulation. It's a simple mnemonic that encapsulates a powerful truth: the primacy of breath. I teach my students that without a clear airway and proper breathing, the intricate systems of the human body falter. It's a reminder that breath is not merely a biological function, but the very essence of life.

Breath holds a spiritual significance as well. It's a gift from the Divine, a breath of life that was first bestowed upon humankind at the dawn of creation. This life-giving breath extends beyond mere existence; it is a call to live fully and abundantly. Our faith teaches us that this isn't where the story ends. The same Creator who breathed life into our first breath also provides us with the Holy Spirit—the divine presence that guides us to reach our highest potential, to blossom and thrive in all aspects of life.

The journey from new mother to nurse and now to mentor has taught me the intricate value of a single breath. It's a continuous reminder that every inhale and exhale is a delicate dance between life and its Creator, between our physical being and our spiritual essence. It is a profound truth I carry with me in both my personal and professional life, a truth I pass on to those I have the privilege to teach.

The Breath of the Holy Spirit

The breath of the Holy Spirit, a profound symbol of life and divine empowerment, not only sustains us but also enriches our lives with an abundance that transcends mere existence. This abundance is vividly articulated in Job's declaration, "For the spirit of God made me, the breath of the Almighty keeps me alive" (Job 33:4). It speaks of a life nurtured by divine breath, one that flourishes under the watchful eye of the Creator.

This divine breath is a testament to the life-giving power of God, who desires life in all its fullness for us. Isaiah 11:1–3 foretold that the Holy Spirit would bestow gifts on the coming Messiah: gifts of wisdom, understanding, counsel, fortitude, knowledge, piety, and fear of the Lord. St. Thomas Aquinas later explored how these same gifts guide us today, embodying traits that foster fullness of life.

Throughout the narratives of the Old Testament, we encounter women who translated these gifts of the Holy Spirit into transformative acts of conviction and courage. Judith was a fearless warrior who met her foe head on. She did not waver when it was time to be present in battle. She called upon the Lord for help.

"So while we wait for the salvation that comes from him,
let us call upon him to help us, and he will hear our cry
if it pleases him."

Judith 8:17

Esther prayed, fasted, and sought counsel from God before intervening for her people. Ruth chose the unknown and practiced obedience over comfort by following her mother-in-law Naomi. The wisdom she received led her to become the great-grandmother of King David! She also foretold the inclusion of the Gentiles in Christ's salvation of His people. Fundamental to these biblical women living these truths was an intimate relationship with God, seeking Him with prayer and trusting in His desire and agency to answer them. They did not doubt their abilities because they did not doubt their God.

Judith's bravery, Esther's wisdom, and Ruth's fidelity are examples of divine gifts in action. Their stories of reliance on God are not distant tales but are echoed in the lived experiences of women today, especially in the journey of motherhood. The same gifts given to these women of the Old Testament are also given to you! The Holy Spirit's breath infuses mothers with the fortitude needed to face each day, the wisdom to make prudent choices for our families, and the understanding to nurture whole health for ourselves and our children.

In the context of self-care, the Holy Spirit's breath is a reminder that caring for oneself is not an act of indulgence but a divine imperative. Self-care is crucial, for it allows women, especially mothers, to replenish their strength, maintain their well-being, and thus better fulfill their vocation of motherhood. It's in the quiet moments of prayer, in the stillness of meditation, and in the restorative practices of self-care that mothers can listen to and feel the guidance of the Holy Spirit. It is here that they are reminded of their worth, empowered to care for their children, and emboldened to advocate for themselves and their families.

Moreover, empowerment in motherhood comes from recognizing the Holy Spirit's gifts within oneself and understanding that these are not just for personal edification but also for nurturing the next generation. Endowed with the breath of life from the Holy Spirit, you are called to be the first teachers of wisdom, the primary counselors of understanding, and enduring examples of piety for your children.

Your God, who breathed life into you, will not leave you wanting for strength or wisdom. Seeking Him allows you to discover the reservoir of divine gifts within, enabling you to approach self-care as a spiritual exercise that equips you to care for your children with greater love, patience, and insight. Asking for His help in finding reliable resources and guidance assures that the care you provide is informed, intentional, and inspired.

Therefore, the breath of the Holy Spirit is not merely a life-giving force but also a source of fortitude and empowerment. It encourages you to embrace the full spectrum of your roles as you journey through the joys and challenges of raising children. With each breath you take, the Holy Spirit offers a reminder of God's enduring presence, a presence that sustains, strengthens, and guides you in the sacred task entrusted to you.

Breathe Intentionally

Taking intentional or deep breaths is a simple yet powerful practice that can benefit you in multiple ways. I used to get perturbed when someone told me to "take a deep breath and calm down!" Then, one day during a challenging shift at work, a fellow nurse asked, "Is holding your breath helping?" Wow! What a mental shift. When I asked myself that question, I realized the negative impact holding my breath and staying upset had on my emotional well-being and cognitive ability.

Deep breathing helps reduce stress, promotes relaxation, and calms the mind. It can enhance mental clarity, increase oxygen intake, and regulate emotions. Through deep breathing exercises, you can relieve anxiety, enhance your ability to cope with challenges, and cultivate a sense of inner peace. This allows you to approach daily tasks with a centered and calm demeanor, enabling you to better handle the demands of motherhood.

How can you make it practical? Techniques that work for me are to ask myself questions, pray a chosen prayer, or to set intentions.

For example:

- **Questions:** How am I feeling now? Is this feeling serving me? How would I rather be feeling? What can I do to direct my thoughts?

- **Prayers:** Jesus taught the apostles the Our Father while He walked on earth (see Matthew 6:9–13). Saying the Our Father slowly, one line at a time, while taking a deep inhale, holding the inhale, exhaling, and holding the exhale is powerful.

- **Intentions:** Say the Jesus Prayer five times, each time offering your day, heart, mind, words, and actions (or whatever makes sense to you) and then again five times, each time receiving His love, mercy, compassion, wisdom, strength (or whatever you need most from Him). The Jesus Prayer is: "Lord Jesus Christ, Son of the living God, have mercy on me, a sinner."

Taking Care of Your Baby's Breath

A normal breathing pattern for babies can vary quite a bit, especially when they are newborns. Here are some general guidelines, but always consult with your pediatrician if you have any concerns about your baby's breathing.

- **Newborns and early infancy** typically breathe thirty to sixty times per minute.

- **Three- to six-month-olds:** As they grow, their breathing rate will slow down to thirty to forty-five breaths per minute.

- **Older infants** (six to twelve months) breathe around twenty-five to forty times per minute.[24]

During the first few months of life, it's normal for infants to breathe somewhat irregularly. They may even take a series of breaths

---

24   "Pediatric Vital Signs: What's Normal and When to Be Concerned," Cleveland Clinic, accessed April 22, 2025, https://health.clevelandclinic.org/pediatric-vital-signs.

followed by a short period of no breathing for five to ten seconds. This is known as periodic breathing.[25] This is usually normal but can be alarming for parents to watch.

Tips and Tricks for Easy Breathing

Babies naturally breathe through their nostrils for the first few months of life. This innate reflex is crucial for effective breastfeeding, as it allows the baby to breathe while sucking and swallowing. Nasal passages in infants are narrower than in older children and adults, making them more susceptible to congestion. If a baby's nose is blocked, it can cause difficulty in feeding and sleeping and may lead to distress. This nose-breathing preference gradually diminishes as babies mature and develop the ability to breathe through their mouths, a transition that provides a safeguard against nasal blockages. Nasal congestion, mucus buildup, and respiratory infections can cause discomfort and difficulty in breathing. However, there are simple techniques that parents and caregivers can employ at home to promote clear nasal passages and facilitate easier breathing. These techniques include using nasal saline, nasal suction, and knowing when to seek medical help for breathing issues. Here are four tips and tricks:

1. **Nasal suction:** Bulb suction (nasal aspirator) is a useful tool for clearing mucus from a child's nose. It is particularly helpful for infants who are unable to blow their noses.

    a. Squeeze the bulb of the suction device and insert the tip gently into the nostril.

    b. Release the bulb slowly to create suction, and then gradually remove the mucus from the nostril.

---

25   American Academy of Pediatrics, "Phases of Sleep: REM and Non-REM Sleep Cycles," HealthyChildren.org, accessed April 22, 2025, https://www.healthychildren.org/English/ages-stages/baby/sleep/Pages/phases-of-sleep.aspx.

  c. Clean the bulb suction thoroughly after each use to prevent the spread of germs.

If using another nasal suction device, follow the package insert directions.

2. **Nasal saline:** Nasal saline solution is a safe and effective way to relieve nasal congestion in children. It helps to moisten the nasal passages, loosen mucus, and facilitate its removal.

  a. Use store-bought nasal saline drops. If you choose to make your own saline, ask your pediatric provider for a recipe and make sure to always use distilled or sterilized water.

  b. Lie your infant on their back or tilt their head back slightly.

  c. Administer two to three drops of saline solution into each nostril.

  d. Allow a few moments for the saline to soften the mucus.

  e. Use a bulb suction or nasal aspirator to gently remove the loosened mucus from the nostrils.

  f. Repeat as necessary, up to three times a day.

3. **Humidifier:** Using a humidifier in the child's bedroom can help add moisture to the air, relieving dry nasal passages and reducing congestion. Ensure that the humidifier is cleaned regularly to prevent the growth of mold or bacteria. Avoid using medications, essential oils, or scented vapors with the humidifier.

4. **Encourage fluid intake:** Staying hydrated can help thin mucus and ease breathing. Encourage your baby to continue breastfeeding or drink their formula but remember that plain water should not be given to an infant under the age of six months. Cleaning their nose out with saline and a bulb suction prior to eating may help them be more comfortable.

Abnormal Breathing

How do I know when my baby's breathing is not normal?

Recognizing signs of abnormal breathing in children is crucial for parents and caregivers to ensure their children's well-being and seek appropriate medical attention when necessary. While occasional variations in breathing patterns are common, persistent or significant abnormalities may indicate an underlying respiratory issue. Here are five signs of abnormal breathing in children to be aware of:

1. **Rapid breathing** (tachypnea): Rapid breathing is characterized by a significantly higher respiratory rate than normal for a child's age. In infants, this can be observed as more than sixty breaths per minute. The best way to assess rapid breathing is to set a timer for one minute, gently place your hand on your baby's chest/stomach, and count the number of breaths. Rapid breathing can be a sign of various respiratory conditions such as pneumonia, asthma, or an obstructed airway. It is essential to monitor for other symptoms like fever, decreased activity or feeds, cough, wheezing, or chest retractions and seek medical attention if rapid breathing persists or is accompanied by concerning symptoms.

2. **Shallow breathing:** Shallow breathing is characterized by reduced depth of each breath, resulting in less air intake. Children with shallow breathing may appear to take quick, shallow breaths rather than deep, regular breaths. Shallow breathing can be caused by respiratory conditions, such as lung diseases or airway obstructions, and may also occur due to pain or anxiety. If shallow breathing persists or is accompanied by other symptoms like cyanosis (bluish discoloration), fussiness, lethargy, decreased feeds or other concerns, prompt medical evaluation is necessary.

3. **Noisy breathing:** Noisy breathing refers to abnormal sounds produced during the breathing process. These sounds can include whistling or squeaky noises when breathing, grunting, or snoring-like noises. Noisy breathing can be caused by various factors, such as respiratory infections, allergies, asthma, or anatomical abnormalities in the airway. If noisy breathing persists, is associated with respiratory distress or rapid breathing, or affects a child's ability to eat, sleep, or babble comfortably, medical evaluation is recommended to determine the underlying cause and provide appropriate treatment.

4. **Irregular breathing:** Irregular breathing patterns involve unpredictable variations in the timing, depth, or rhythm of breaths. Examples include periods of apnea (temporary pauses in breathing) or episodes of rapid, shallow breaths followed by slower, deeper breaths. Irregular breathing can be a sign of respiratory disorders like sleep apnea, respiratory distress syndrome, or central nervous system abnormalities. If irregular breathing patterns are observed frequently or are accompanied by other concerning symptoms like lethargy, poor feeding, or color changes, medical attention should be sought.

5. **Labored breathing:** Labored breathing, also known as respiratory distress, is characterized by increased effort and discomfort during breathing. Signs of labored breathing include retractions (visible pulling in of the muscles between the ribs or at the base of the neck), flaring nostrils, grunting sounds, or the use of accessory muscles (e.g., neck or abdominal muscles) to assist breathing. Labored breathing can indicate respiratory conditions such as infection, asthma, or other severe conditions. It is crucial to seek immediate medical attention if your child shows signs of labored breathing, since it can be a medical emergency requiring prompt intervention.

If any signs of abnormal breathing are observed in your child, it is important to remain calm and seek medical advice. Additional warning signs to watch for include sweating on the head or cool, clammy skin, a barking or incessant cough, and high-pitched sounds or gasping for air. Remember that every baby is different, and what's normal for one may not be for another. If you're ever unsure about your baby's breathing patterns, it's best to consult with a healthcare professional.

Contacting a healthcare professional or visiting an emergency department can help assess the severity of the condition, identify the underlying cause, and initiate appropriate treatment. Emergent medical evaluation (calling 911) is particularly necessary if the child's breathing difficulty is severe, or accompanied by other alarming symptoms like high fever, chest pain, or altered consciousness.

Trust your instincts and seek medical evaluation when you are concerned about your child's breathing patterns. Early detection and appropriate management of abnormal breathing is crucial for ensuring the best possible health outcomes.

The Gift of Breath

God breathed life into you and your little one. He also gave you the Holy Spirit who wants to breathe His gifts into you. The Spirit wants to help you understand how to grow spiritually so that you are of sound mind to make decisions for yourself and your child.

The Holy Spirit provides spiritual breath for mothers, filling them with strength, wisdom, and comfort in their journey of motherhood. Through His presence, we find the patience to nurture, the discernment to make decisions, and the love to care for our children. The Holy Spirit breathes life into our weary souls, helping us navigate the joys and challenges of motherhood with grace and reliance on God's guidance.

Trust the Holy Spirit as you care for your infant. He will give you wisdom to know when to use simple techniques at home to promote easy breathing for children such as using nasal saline, nasal aspiration, and a humidifier when needed. The Holy Spirit can also help you discern when to seek medical help if breathing difficulties persist, worsen, or are accompanied by severe symptoms. Consulting a healthcare professional with any persistent or severe breathing concerns ensures appropriate evaluation and care. Through it all, remember that every breath your child takes is a gift from God and He will guide you in protecting your infant.

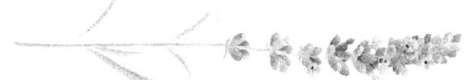

READ: *"Send forth your spirit, they are created and you renew the face of the earth."* (Psalm 104:30)

MEDITATE: Envision yourself welcoming the Holy Spirit to be present with you and come into your heart.

PRAY: Come, Holy Spirit, fill the hearts of your faithful
and kindle in them the fire of your love.
Send forth your Spirit and they shall be created,
and you shall renew the face of the earth.

Let us pray.
O God, who have taught the hearts of the faithful
by the light of the Holy Spirit,
grant that in the same Spirit we may be truly wise
and ever rejoice in his consolation.
Through Christ our Lord. Amen.[26]

LISTEN: "Come Holy Spirit" by Coffey Anderson

RESOLVE: While praying the prayer to the Holy Spirit, practice intentional breathing exercises.

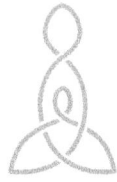

---

26   "Prayer to the Holy Spirit," *USCCB*, https://www.usccb.org/prayers/prayer-holy-spirit.

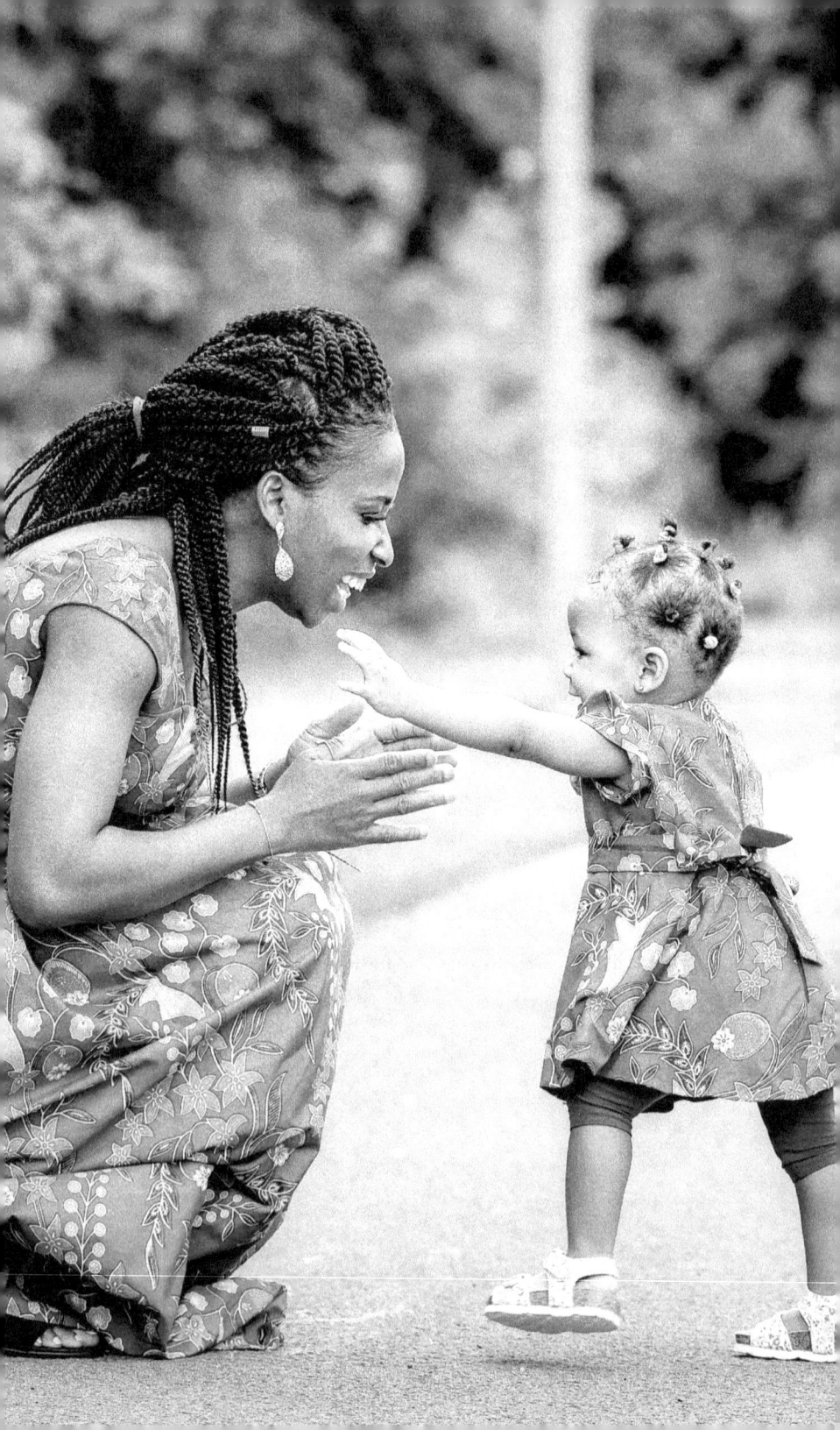

CHAPTER 5

Nourishment to Grow and Thrive

"And for this reason we too give thanks to God unceasingly, that, in receiving the word of God from hearing us, you received not a human word but, as it truly is, the word of God, which is now at work in you who believe."

—1 Thessalonians 2:13

As we discussed in the last chapter, God breathed the breath of life and the power of the Holy Spirit into each of us. God's Spirit dwells within us, granting us patience, love, and wisdom as we navigate the challenges of raising children. God's desire is for our whole health to be nurtured by Him.

Throughout the Bible, we are reminded of God's desire to provide for His children. God's love and care are demonstrated throughout Scripture. He is eager to nourish and sustain each of us with His unconditional love and the truth of His word.

His word is alive in each of us, nourishing, guiding, and working. God calls us to seek Him and His truth as our spiritual food so we can live according to His will. God's love and grace provide strength for the physical, emotional, and spiritual demands of motherhood. His Word offers wisdom and guidance, reminding us of our invaluable worth and purpose. He provides us with support and encouragement, reminding us we are not alone in our journey of motherhood. God often provides small blessings and unexpected moments of grace that bring joy and renewal to our weary hearts and bodies. Ultimately, God sustains and nourishes us by offering His unfailing love and reminding us that our labors of love are valuable and eternally significant.

In the physical realm, God's provision is evident in His creation. From the vastness of the universe to the intricacy of the human body, every detail reflects His careful design. In the book of Psalms, King David writes, "The eyes of all look hopefully to you; you give them their food in due season. You open wide your hand and satisfy the desire of every living thing" (Psalm 145:15–16).

The Bible describes numerous occasions when God physically nourished his people in times of need. When the Israelites wandered hungry in the desert after their exodus from Egypt, God provided manna, which sustained them for forty years until they reached the Promised Land. In 1 Kings, during a devastating famine, God miraculously sustained the widow of Zarephath, the prophet Elijah, and her son by ensuring her jar of flour and jug of oil never ran empty. Perhaps most famously, Jesus himself fed multitudes with just five loaves and two fish, with twelve baskets of leftovers remaining. These stories beautifully illustrate God's role as the ultimate Provider, meeting the needs of all His children. Just as we ensure our children have enough to eat, God desires to nourish and sustain us.

Beyond physical nourishment, God is also concerned with our emotional well-being. In the Gospel of Matthew, Jesus reminds His followers of God's care for them, saying, "Therefore I tell you, do not worry about your life, what you will eat, or about your body, what you will wear. Is not life more than food and the body more than clothing? Look at the birds in the sky; they do not sow or reap, they gather nothing into barns, yet your heavenly Father feeds them. Are not you more important than they?" (Matthew 6:25–26). These verses highlight God's intimate knowledge of our needs and His desire for us to trust in Him completely. By recognizing His provision for the birds in the air, we can find assurance that God will also provide for us.

The nourishment and sustenance God offers extend beyond the physical and emotional realms. God's ultimate desire is for us to be spiritually nourished and fulfilled. In the Gospel of John, Jesus proclaims, "I am the bread of life; whoever comes to me will never hunger, and whoever believes in me will never thirst" (John 6:35). These powerful words illustrate that true satisfaction and sustenance can only be found in a relationship with God through Jesus Christ. By accepting His love and grace, we are spiritually nourished and sustained for eternity.

Throughout history, the saints demonstrated how God's sustaining love nourished not only them but those they served. St. Catherine of Siena, a renowned fourteenth-century mystic, deeply embraced the concept of God's love as her ultimate source of spiritual nourishment and sustenance. Her commitment to serving the poor and tending to the sick in hospitals was an extension of this belief, and she saw each act of charity as feeding the soul with God's compassion. Catherine's life and writings illustrate how being fed by divine love enables us to feed others through acts of giving and caring. St. Catherine likened God's love to mother's milk and prayed we would accept the nourishment from Him.

"Dearest sister in Jesus. I, Catherine, servant of the servants of Jesus, write to you in His Precious Blood, wishing only that you feed yourself with God's love and nourish yourself with it as at a mother's breast. Nobody in fact can live without this milk!"[27]

God desires to meet our physical, emotional, and spiritual needs. As we lean on Him and trust in His promises, we can find true satisfaction and fulfillment. All mothers should remember that God's nourishment and sustenance are freely offered to us, inviting us into a relationship that brings abundant life and eternal purpose. With His love working in us, we are able to reflect His love to our children. Through our love as mothers, we provide a foundation of confidence, resilience, and love, enabling our children to navigate life's challenges. Below are some practical tips for taking care of yourself and your little one.

Mother's Self-Care

Feeding an infant is a full-time endeavor! Your own nourishment is essential to your infant's well-being. Whether you are formula feeding or breastfeeding, you must have proper nutrition for your body to recover from pregnancy, heal from childbirth, and have the energy and stamina needed to care for your infant.

Embrace a diet rich in nutrients and hydration. Foods like leafy greens, lean proteins, whole grains, and fruits are not only beneficial for milk production but also vital for replenishing your body. When friends or family members asked what they could do to help, I told them to bring dinner. An important part of the request was that it did not have to be homemade. I also created baskets for snacks and water and placed them throughout the house. One was by the nursing chair and another by my bed. When I got up to use the

---

27   Catherine of Siena, *The Letters of Saint Catherine of Siena*, vatican.va, https://www.vatican.va/spirit/documents/spirit_20010814_caterina-siena_en.html.

restroom, nurse the baby, or pump, I drank a bottle of water and ate a snack. My husband wanted to help me but felt like he could not do much since I was breastfeeding, so he kept the baskets filled with supplies. This proved to be so helpful to keep my milk supply flowing and give me the energy I needed.

- **Tune into your body's needs** and the tender moments with your baby, creating a balance that fosters both physical health and emotional well-being. Here are some helpful tips:

- **Rest and rejuvenate:** Rest is not a luxury; it is a necessity. Sleep or rest when your baby sleeps. These stolen moments of rest can be deeply rejuvenating. The demands of laundry and dishes are ever present. What helped me was to intentionally lie down every other time my baby did. The times in between I would dedicate to getting household chores done. Even brief naps (ten to twenty minutes) can help repair and restore your energy levels. If you get on social media, set a timer for yourself and then put your phone down. There were times that I was breastfeeding or lying down to rest and before I knew it, thirty minutes were lost in the world of social media. I started setting a timer for three to ten minutes, and then I would put the phone away. This freed up my mind and time to be fully present with my baby or to rest.

- **Surround yourself** with a supportive community, whether family, friends, or breastfeeding support groups. Sharing experiences, concerns, and joys is uplifting and informative. Remember, asking for help is not a sign of weakness but of strength and wisdom.

- **Embrace the little moments** by mindfully being with your baby. You know the chaotic moments will occur, so intentionally pause during the sweet moments to fill your cup. Breathe in their sweet scent after bath time, rub your cheek on their soft head when carrying them, or cherish the motion of rocking as you calm their cries. These moments of mindfulness amid the whirlwind of motherhood are grounding and calming.

- **Physical activity** is as important as eating and sleeping. Honor your unique, divinely created body and commit to movement every day. Even light activities like a short walk or ten minutes of restorative stretching can make a significant, positive impact. As you recover from childbirth or a C-section, you can increase your movement according to your healthcare provider's recommendations. Being a mom is an unrecognized sport! Movement will help keep your muscles engaged, your body functioning at its best, and provide a mental uplift.

- **Invest in a good breastfeeding pillow.** It will provide support during nursing, bottle feeding, or holding your baby by helping to reduce strain on your arms, shoulders, and neck. The support can help your entire upper body, including breast discomfort. I suffered from carpal tunnel syndrome as a result of lifting and holding my nine-plus-pound babies. Breastfeeding pillows may also be used when holding a baby to prevent fatigue. Please remember, however, that these pillows should never be used to prop infants while sleeping. Additionally, babies should never be left unattended while playing around a pillow or propped on a breastfeeding pillow.

- **Celebrate!** Even a seemingly small win can be joyfully experienced with a smile or little happy dance! Your body, mind, and spirit are growing and changing you into a beautiful mother! Give glory to God and rejoice!

Remember that self-care is not just a series of actions; it is a mindset. It is giving yourself permission to prioritize your well-being, understanding that by caring for yourself, you are creating a reservoir of strength and love from which both you and your baby will deeply benefit.

Breast Milk and Formula

Feeding a baby provides a rich opportunity to meet their whole health needs. It provides an opportunity to foster connections that encourage bonding, security, and affection. This lays the groundwork for the infant's future emotional health and social relationships. The decision to breastfeed or formula feed is a very personal choice and may be different for each family.

Regardless of whether you breastfeed or use formula, early skin-to-skin contact is crucial to the emotional connection with your baby and helps release hormones that aid in the transition from pregnancy to motherhood. When my first son was born, the first thing the lactation consultant did was take my baby out of his blanket and onesie, leaving him only in a diaper, and then place him directly on my chest. I thought she was going to teach him to latch, but instead she told us to just rest together, that we had both traveled an exhausting journey of childbirth and we needed to hold each other. My heart was overwhelmed by this intimate, physical expression of love. When he was resting on my chest, I could feel my breasts begin to fill with colostrum. Being skin-to-skin with your baby encourages a natural release of the hormone oxytocin that stimulates milk production and promotes a sense of calm for us moms. Love filled my heart and entire being. My husband's job was to watch over both of us; if I started to fall asleep, he was to put our son safely in his bassinet. I was soon able to nurse my son. The memory of this time was imprinted in my mind and heart and helped me when I had my second baby. Holding him close to me was very powerful.

While I chose to breastfeed both of my sons, I didn't frown upon the use of formula. After the birth of my second son via C-section, his blood sugar was dangerously low. This was due to a complication of my insulin-dependent diabetes. I was given the choice to send him directly to the neonatal intensive care unit (NICU) or have the nurses in the operating room offer him a bottle of formula. My husband and I decided he would be given a bottle of formula. While my milk was coming in, we did need to supplement with formula for a few days. Sometimes you will hear women talk about using donated breast milk from a family member or friend or giving their own breast milk to others. Before deciding to use or donate milk to family or friends, however, recognize there can be health risks involved, particularly related to infectious diseases. Anyone who is considering using donated milk should discuss the risks and benefits with their primary care provider and should take time to carefully discern this decision.

Breast milk is regarded as the gold standard for infant nutrition. It's a complete source of nutrition, rich in antibodies, enzymes, and nutrients that support optimal growth and development. Breastfeeding offers numerous benefits for your infant, including a reduced risk of respiratory and gastrointestinal infections and allergies. Long-term, breastfeeding is associated with a decreased risk of various conditions such as obesity, diabetes, asthma, some childhood leukemia, and SIDS.[28] Breastfeeding may even lead to better cognitive outcomes, such as higher IQ and improved school performance. It also promotes bonding between mother and child and provides emotional and psychological benefits for both. For mothers, breastfeeding aids in postpartum recovery by helping the uterus contract and reduces bleeding. It's also linked to reduced rates of breast and ovarian cancer, type 2 diabetes, and heart disease, while facilitating weight loss and enhancing emotional health.[29] If you breastfeed, continue to take your prenatal vitamins to ensure you

---

[28] "Breastfeeding Benefits," CDC.gov. Accessed April 23, 2025. https://www.cdc.gov/breastfeeding/features/breastfeeding-benefits.html. See also S.H. Søegaard, M.M. Andersen, K. Rostgaard, et al, "Exclusive Breastfeeding Duration and Risk of Childhood Cancers," *JAMA Network Open*, 2024 Mar 4;7(3):e243115.

[29] American Academy of Pediatrics, "Why Breastfeed?" *HealthyChildren.org*, accessed April 23, 2025, https://www.healthychildren.org/English/ages-stages/baby/breastfeeding/Pages/Why-Breastfeed.aspx.

get the nutrients and vitamins essential to your body's health and wellness.

Though breastfeeding has many benefits, it may present challenges such as difficulties with latching, inadequate milk supply, or discomfort for the mother. Additionally, it requires time, commitment, and support. Ask for a lactation consultant to help you as soon as you are admitted to the hospital. This will help to ensure they come to your aid promptly. Sometimes, however, the in-hospital lactation consults are not enough. With my second son, I needed help after we were home from the hospital. He wasn't gaining weight, and I was experiencing discomfort with cracked and bleeding nipples. I arranged a home visit with a lactation consultant, and she was able to teach both of us how to properly breastfeed. With time and persistence, we both benefitted! Though there are many recommendations for breastfeeding, here are a few tips I suggest:

- Make sure your entire areola is in your baby's mouth.

- Completely empty one breast before having your baby feed on the other breast.

- Do what works for you to remember when feeding times are, how long they last, and which breast you started and ended with. Some moms like journaling, others put a hair tie on their wrist, and some moms use an app. Even a colored bra pad could indicate the breast that is next for feeding!

Formula serves as a suitable alternative when breastfeeding is not possible. Infant formula is carefully formulated to mimic the composition of breast milk, providing essential nutrients necessary for a baby's growth. It's an option for mothers who are unable to breastfeed due to medical conditions, individual circumstances, or personal choice. Formula feeding lacks the immunological properties of breast milk, though, and may not offer the same long-term health benefits. There are also considerations regarding the cost, preparation, and potential for allergies or sensitivities.

Bottle feeding with breast milk or formula allows for others to be involved and offers flexibility. Bonding can still flourish as you hold your baby during the feeding period. Propping the bottle is not advised because of the risk of choking, breathing milk into their lungs, tooth decay, and ear infections.

The choice between breast milk and formula is a personal one that should be made based on prayer, careful consideration of information, individual circumstances, and consulting with healthcare professionals. The most important aspect is ensuring that infants receive adequate nutrition, love, and care to support their healthy development. Whether breastfeeding or formula feeding, what matters most is the well-being and happiness of both the baby and the mother.

Breastfeeding Help for Mama

Nipple and breast pain can be a common challenge for breastfeeding mothers, but fortunately, there are several products and remedies available to help alleviate discomfort. Here are some options:

- **Nipple creams and ointments:** These are specifically designed for breastfeeding mothers (lanolin or vegan options are available).

- **Hydrogel pads:** These pads provide cooling relief and can help soothe sore nipples. They can be placed in the refrigerator for extra cooling effect. These were a saving grace for me. Use *after* your milk has come in. Some help the skin heal faster.

- **Breast shells:** These are worn inside your bra to protect sore nipples from friction and to help ease engorgement by applying gentle pressure.

- **Nursing pads:** Soft, absorbent pads can be placed inside your bra to protect your clothing from milk leakage, which can cause your skin to break down if it remains wet.

- **Warm/cold compresses:** Warm compresses can help stimulate milk flow and relieve engorgement, while cold compresses can reduce swelling and alleviate pain. Use cold compresses after feeds to minimize impact on milk supply.

- **Supportive nursing bra:** A well-fitted, supportive nursing bra can reduce breast pain by providing proper support.

- **Breast pumps:** Using a high-quality, properly fitted breast pump can help if nipple pain is due to latching issues. If you have to pump a lot, consider buying a hands-free pumping bra; it is definitely worth every penny!

- **Manual expression techniques:** Learning and applying manual milk expression techniques can help relieve engorgement and reduce discomfort.

- **Salt water rinse:** A simple saline solution can be used to rinse or soak the nipples after feeding, which can aid in healing sore or cracked nipples.

Talk to your healthcare provider if you experience ongoing challenges or signs of infection such as severe redness and swelling accompanied by fever, chills, and general malaise (similar to flu-like symptoms).

Does My Baby Need Other Vitamins?

Breastfeeding provides most of the nutrients a baby needs, but there are a few exceptions where supplemental vitamins are recommended:

- **Vitamin D:** Breast milk may not provide enough vitamin D, which is essential for bone health. The American Academy of Pediatrics (AAP) recommends a daily vitamin D supplement of 400 IU for all breastfed infants starting soon after birth even if Mom is taking a supplement herself.

- **Iron:** Breast milk contains iron, but not always enough for infants four months of age and older. The AAP advises iron supplements starting at four months for exclusively breastfed infants until iron-rich foods are introduced into their diet.

- **Fluoride:** After six months, if the water supply is deficient in fluoride, a supplement may be recommended by your pediatrician.

How to Select a Formula

If you choose to formula feed, selecting the right formula is crucial for your baby's nutrition. Consult with your pediatrician, who can recommend a formula based on your baby's health and nutritional requirements. Babies with special dietary needs, such as a cow's milk allergy, may require specialized formulas. Your pediatrician can advise on hypoallergenic or other specialized options if needed.

It's also important to understand the ingredients in baby formulas. Most are cow's milk-based with added nutrients, but some have additional components like prebiotics or probiotics. Discuss any additives with your pediatrician to ensure they are necessary or beneficial for your baby. Consider the practical aspects, too, such as preparation and storage. Powdered formulas are economical and have a longer shelf life, while liquid concentrates are easier to prepare. Ready-to-use formulas offer convenience but at a higher cost.

Finally, monitor your baby's reaction to any new formula. Signs of intolerance, such as fussiness, gas, or allergic reactions, should be discussed with a pediatrician, who may suggest a different formula.

High-quality formula can support your baby's growth and health effectively, even though it doesn't exactly match breast milk. With your pediatrician's help, you can find a suitable formula to nourish your baby.

What about Water, Juice, and Other Liquids?

For the first six months of life, your infant only needs breast milk or formula unless otherwise directed by your healthcare provider for a specific reason.

Plain water should not be given to an infant younger than six months because their kidneys aren't developed enough. After six months old, you may start to offer four to eight ounces of plain water per day.[30]

Other than breast milk, formula, and then water after six months of age, your infant doesn't need any other type of liquids. You may hear of people offering fruit juice to infants. While this is a popular solution to introducing fruits, juice contains a high sugar content and does not have the same nutrients contained in pureed or whole fruits. Nutritionally, babies do not need juice.[31] We recommend delaying the introduction of juice for as long as possible. Occasionally, prune or apple juice may be recommended for constipation. You can offer it watered down in a 1:1 ratio, but you should talk to your pediatric provider first before using this as a treatment method.

Introducing Solids

The transition from breast milk or formula to solid foods is an exciting milestone in a baby's development. This transition represents a significant shift in your baby's nutritional journey and marks the beginning of their exploration of new tastes and textures. The following are some guidelines for the best way to introduce solid foods to babies:

---

30   American Academy of Pediatrics, "Recommended Drinks for Young Children Ages 0–5,"
      HealthyChildren.org, accessed April 23, 2025, https://www.healthychildren.org/English/healthy-living/
      nutrition/Pages/recommended-drinks-for-young-children-ages-0-5.aspx.

31   American Academy of Pediatrics, "Recommended Drinks for Young Children Ages 0–5."

- **Timing:** The American Academy of Pediatrics recommends exclusive breastfeeding for the first six months of a baby's life. Around the age of six months, babies are typically developmentally ready for solid foods. Look for signs of readiness, such as sitting up with support, showing interest in food, and being able to move food to the back of their mouth.

- **Taste buds and window of opportunity:** Babies are born with a natural inclination toward sweet flavors, an evolutionary trait likely developed to ensure the appeal of breast milk. However, as they grow and start exploring solid foods, their taste buds, which are more sensitive than those of adults, begin to shape their food preferences. During this important stage, introducing a variety of flavors and textures is essential in developing a well-rounded palate. Early exposure to fruits, vegetables, and whole grains can guide infants' taste buds towards preferring these nutritious options over high-sugar alternatives. By offering a wide range of wholesome foods, you can lay a strong foundation for your child's long-term health and dietary choices.

- **Start with single foods:** When introducing solid foods, start with single pureed or mashed vegetables or fruits. The American Academy of Pediatrics recommends starting one food every three to five days.[32] This allows you to identify any potential allergies or sensitivities and helps the baby become familiar with individual flavors. Foods considered to be allergenic should be introduced before age one for optimal tolerance. If you have a family history of food allergies, discuss introducing these foods with your healthcare provider prior to

---

32   American Academy of Pediatrics, "Starting Solid Foods," *HealthyChildren.org*, accessed February 13, 2025, https://www.healthychildren.org/English/ages-stages/baby/feeding-nutrition/Pages/Starting-Solid-Foods.aspx.

introducing them.[33] If you have any concerns about allergic reactions to new foods you have given your infant (hives, facial swelling, breathing difficulties, vomiting), contact your provider immediately.

KATHRYN

Sometimes I think God has a sense of humor. As an outpatient pediatrician, I saw countless patients with food allergies. During my first pregnancy, I distinctly remember thinking, *I hope my daughter does not have any food allergies.* When we began to introduce solid foods, everything seemed initially fine. However, just before her first birthday, she had several reactions to baked goods containing eggs. Though initially I hoped it was a fluke, allergy testing confirmed not only an egg allergy but also a severe peanut allergy.

Our initial disappointment and anxiety quickly gave way to a new normal. We eliminated all peanut products from our house, and I began experimenting with egg-free recipes. I quickly learned how to make excellent-tasting eggless baked goods!

And while it would not have been the path I would have chosen, I discovered that this diagnosis helped me relate to my patients more. I developed genuine empathy for families navigating food allergies. I also became more attuned to atypical allergy symptoms since my daughter's reactions manifested as lethargy and vomiting, not the typical rash or hives. Understanding her reactions and receiving her diagnosis made me a better pediatrician.

After discovering a fabulous chocolate cake recipe that was both egg- and dairy-free, I even started printing copies of it to give to patients if the subject came up. If a parent was worried about having to find a cake recipe to make for a birthday or celebration, I would offer them the recipe. To this day, it is the most requested recipe my children ask for on their birthdays. You can find the recipe in Appendix 5, and I hope you enjoy it as much as we do!

---

33   E .M. Abrams, M. Shaker M, D. Stukus, D.P. Mack, M. Greenhawt, "Updates in Food Allergy Prevention in Children," *Pediatrics*, 2023 Nov 1;152(5):e2023062836.

- **Texture progression:** As your baby becomes accustomed to pureed foods, gradually introduce thicker textures and mashed or finely chopped foods. This helps them develop their chewing and swallowing skills. Eventually, they can transition to soft finger foods and more varied textures—typically between eight to nine months old when they develop a "pincer grasp."

- **Maintain a safe feeding environment:** Always supervise your baby during feeding times and ensure they are seated upright to reduce the risk of choking. Avoid offering foods that are choking hazards, such as whole grapes, nuts, or large chunks of food. Cut foods into small, pea-sized pieces.

- **Be patient, persistent, and enjoy!** Introducing solid foods is a gradual process. It can take several tries for babies to develop a liking for certain flavors. Keep offering foods multiple times, even if they initially reject them. Make feeding times a pleasant and interactive experience by sitting together, offering encouragement, and allowing them to explore and play with their food. If possible, have the entire family eat at least one meal at the same time your baby eats. Be willing to embrace

WHAT ABOUT BABY-LED WEANING?

Baby-led weaning (BLW) is a popular approach to introducing solid foods in which babies are encouraged to self-feed using their hands rather than being spoon-fed purees. Advocates of BLW suggest it promotes independence, improves hand-eye coordination, and allows babies to explore different textures and flavors at their own pace. However, some healthcare providers have been concerned about the risk of choking, potential for insufficient iron and other nutrient intake, and inadequate weight gain among babies being fed by a pure BLW technique. While some research has indicated that these concerns may not be warranted, overall there is a lack of high-quality data about the true benefits of BLW compared with traditional feeding methods. Thus far, studies indicate that aside from possible social benefits, BLW is not significantly better than traditional feeding methods in terms of safety or nutrition.[34]

One of the larger studies on the topic, commonly referred to as the BLISS study (Baby-Led Introduction to SolidS), measured outcomes in families who used a modified version of BLW to address some of the concerns raised by healthcare providers. In this version, parents received proper education about feeding their infants and were instructed to offer at least three different foods per meal, including one that was iron-rich and one that was higher in calories. This approach suggests that the overall safety and nutritional outcomes of BLW may depend significantly on how it is practiced, rather than BLW itself being inherently superior to traditional methods.[35]

If you choose to practice a form of BLW, know that it is absolutely acceptable (and sometimes necessary) to supplement with spoon-fed purees, which can provide important nutrients like iron and healthy fats in a safer, easier-to-consume form. A combined approach may offer the best of both worlds. The goal is to offer a variety of foods that support your baby's growth and development, while also keeping safety and nutrition as the priority.

---

34   E. D'Auria, M. Bergamini, A. Staiano, et al, Italian Society of Pediatrics, "Baby-Led Weaning: What a Systematic Review of the Literature Adds On," Italian Journal of Pediatrics, 2018 May 3;44(1):49.

35   L. Daniels, R. W. Taylor, S.M. Williams, et al, "Impact of a Modified Version of Baby-Led Weaning on Iron Intake and Status: A Randomised Controlled Trial," BMJ Open, 2018 Jun 27;8(6):e019036.

some mess and have fun learning with your baby.

In Summary

As we meet the nutritional demands of our own bodies and our child's, God wants us to know He is ever present. His love and the truth of His Word are always available. God's sustenance surpasses physical nourishment, focusing also on our emotional and spiritual well-being. This aspect is particularly significant in motherhood, where we encounter diverse challenges and responsibilities. In our relationship with God, we can find strength and wisdom, equipping us to navigate the complexities and joys of raising children.

Throughout the Bible, God's intent to holistically nourish His people is clear. He invites us to partake in a life enriched with His knowledge and love. This invitation is deeply intertwined with the essence of motherhood, where nurturing life becomes a profound expression of living out God's truth. We have the great gift of reflecting God's selfless love and care, embracing God's desire for us to thrive in His nourishment and ultimately share in eternal life with Him.

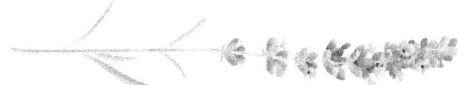

READ: *"Jesus said to them, 'I am the bread of life; whoever comes to me will never hunger, and whoever believes in me will never thirst.'"* (John 6:35)

MEDITATE: Close your eyes and imagine yourself sitting at the table of the Lord. You are weary and aware of your imperfections, yet He welcomes you with tender love. Envision God offering you nourishment—not just bread for your body, but truth for your mind and love for your soul.

PRAY: Holy Spirit, come into my heart;
draw it to Thee by Thy power, O my God,
and grant me charity with filial fear.
Preserve me, O beautiful Love, from every evil thought;
warm me, inflame me with Thy dear love,
and every pain will seem light to me.
My Father, my sweet Lord, help me in all my actions.
Jesus, love, Jesus, love. Amen.[36]

LISTEN: "Bigger Table" by Matt Maher

RESOLVE:
1. Choose a Bible verse that feeds you the truth of God's love. Write it down to memorize or look at throughout your day.
2. Write the ways, both big and small, the Lord has fed you and nourished you over the past several months.

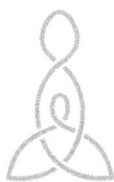

---

36   St. Catherine of Siena, "Come into My Heart," Ascension Press, accessed June 9, 2025, https://ascensionpress.com/pages/st-catherine-of-siena.

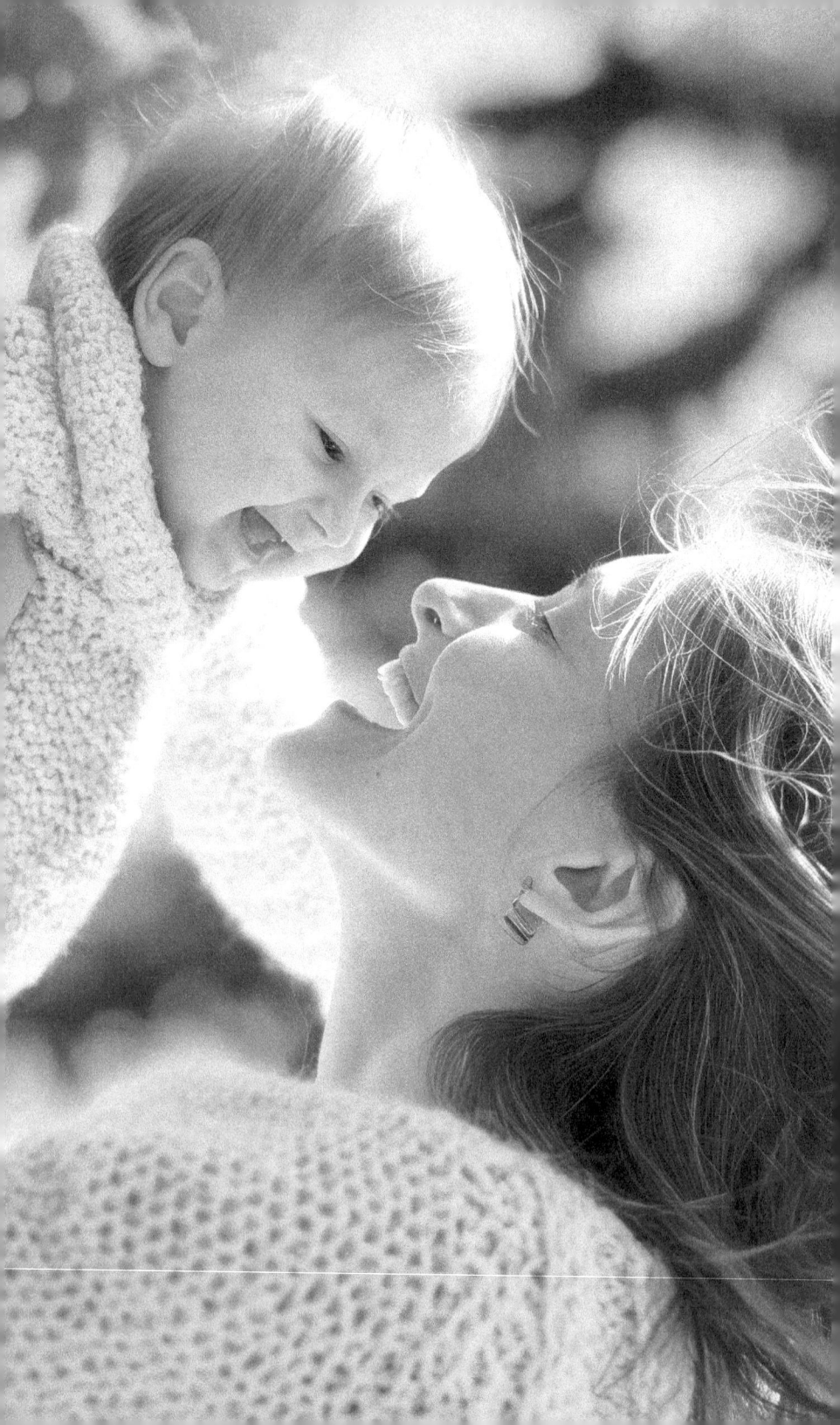

CHAPTER 6

The Gut Feeling and Your Baby's Belly

As a nurse, I often received the advice to "trust your gut." This intuitive sense, while valuable, is not solely based on instinct. It's an accumulation of years of training, knowledge, and experience. Recognizing a patient's deterioration before vital signs change is not just intuition but a skill honed through diligent practice and observation.

As I transitioned into motherhood, the same advice also surfaced: "Trust your mommy gut." Despite the plethora of parenting books, videos, conversations with pediatricians, and my own knowledge as a pediatric nurse practitioner, I still experienced moments of doubt and insecurity. At these moments, I realized that my humanness was insufficient and I needed to practice seeking guidance from the Holy Spirit.

"Trust in the Lord with all your heart, on your own intelligence do not rely; In all your ways be mindful of Him, and He will make straight your paths."

—Proverbs 3:5–6

The beautiful truth is that He always showed up. From large decisions about seeking healthcare to smaller choices such as introducing sweet potatoes or green beans first, guidance from the Holy Spirit was readily available. I had to humble myself, accept that I didn't have all the answers, and then seek help through prayer and discernment. This was really tested for my husband and me when our younger son was only two weeks old. During a diaper change, I recognized the telltale signs of a skin infection that would require antibiotics. I knew the possibility of hospitalization and intravenous antibiotic was high, but he was so well appearing that I hesitated to jump to the most aggressive treatment option. The first pediatrician we chose wanted us to go to the emergency room. While I did not think this was unreasonable, I knew in my heart we could try managing the infection at home with oral antibiotics and topical skincare, so we sought a second opinion. After examining our son in the clinic, a new pediatrician agreed completely with a trial of oral antibiotics and a strict cleaning regimen with topical treatment as well. Our intuition was correct, and we felt grateful the pediatrician heard our ideas and stayed in close communication with us. The treatment plan at home was rigorous, but we were grateful to not be in the hospital. Our son did well, and in a few days we saw him turn the corner and heal.

While our human instincts can serve us well, they may not be perfect. Relying solely on our own understanding and human wisdom may lead to confusion and misdirection. This is where discernment through the Holy Spirit becomes essential. As a member of the Trinity, the Holy Spirit imparts gifts of wisdom, knowledge, intuition, love, and peace. These gifts are of divine origin, intended to guide us as we walk in this fallen world. The divine presence dwells within us believers, offering guidance, comfort, and wisdom. Through the Holy Spirit, anyone who asks will receive direction and understanding in navigating the complexities and unpredictable journey of motherhood. This guidance can manifest in various ways, bringing peace in stressful situations and offering insight as we make choices for our children's well-being.

When our gut instinct signals concern, we should turn to the Holy Spirit for guidance. To strengthen our discernment process, we must cultivate a close relationship with God through prayer, study of His Word, and a willingness to listen.

Mary Magdalene exemplifies this commitment to prayer and trust in Jesus. She faithfully walked with Jesus and chose to have a close relationship with Him. She accepted His healing and sought His friendship. Jesus trusted her as the first person to see Him after the Resurrection. Jesus sent the Holy Spirit to Mary Magdalene and prompted her to seek Jesus and recognize Him when He revealed Himself to her. The Holy Spirit then empowered her to spread the good news to the frightened disciples. In each of her choices, Mary Magdalene shows us how the Holy Spirit's presence provides a beacon of hope and clarity.

Seeking the Holy Spirit and trusting our discernment is an essential aspect of our whole health. This guidance is not limited to monumental life choices but is present in our everyday decision-making. We are encouraged to trust in the Lord and submit ourselves to His guidance. By doing so, we open ourselves up to the leading of the Holy Spirit, who can provide clarity and insight beyond our limited perspective.

Trusting the discernment process can be challenging at times, especially when faced with difficult decisions or conflicting advice. However, Jesus promised He would send the Holy Spirit to remind us of the truths of His love, peace, and constant care.

"The Advocate, the Holy Spirit that the Father will send in my name—He will teach everything and remind you of all that [I] told you."

—John 14:26

The Holy Spirit speaks to our hearts, enlightens our minds, and empowers us to make choices that honor God and align with His purposes. God calls us to a mindset of humility, surrendering our own desires and preconceived notions and being open to God's leading.

When discerning God's will, it is crucial to maintain a delicate balance between humility and confidence. Humility enables us to recognize our limited understanding and submit ourselves to God's guidance, while confidence empowers us to trust in His faithfulness and step forward with assurance. These two qualities work hand in hand to help us navigate the complexities of discernment.

James 4:10 reminds us of the importance of humility in our relationship with God, stating, "Humble yourselves before the Lord and he will exalt you." This verse highlights the need to approach God with a humble heart, acknowledging that our wisdom and understanding are limited compared to His. Humility opens the door for us to seek God's will with a teachable spirit, recognizing that we are dependent on His guidance.

Maintaining both humility and confidence requires a deep reliance on God's sovereignty and a willingness to surrender our own desires and agendas. It means seeking God's will with a humble heart, recognizing that His ways are higher than our way, while also trusting in His promises and having confidence in His guidance.

In the process of discerning God's will, humility keeps us from being driven by our own pride or desires, allowing us to remain open to correction and redirection. It reminds us that we are fallible and need God's wisdom to guide us. On the other hand, confidence in God's faithfulness encourages us to move forward with assurance, knowing that He will provide the necessary guidance and equip us for the path ahead. Humility keeps us open and receptive to God's guidance, while confidence allows us to act boldly on that guidance.

Together, they form a dynamic and balanced approach to living a life led by the Holy Spirit, marked by both dependence on God and active engagement with the world. Mother Mary and Jesus are perfect examples of living this life with great humility and confidence.

Food and Eating Patterns Are Full of the Opinions of Others

One area where parents are often required to reflect and discern about what is best for their child involves food and eating choices. Children's food and eating patterns can generate diverse opinions among family members and others. Everyone wants what is best for the child's health and well-being, but conflicting viewpoints can make decision-making challenging. It's important to recognize that food and eating habits play a significant role in a child's growth, development, and overall health. For certain specific topics about food and eating there truly is more than one "correct" way of doing things. However, the opinions of family members and others should be evaluated in light of evidence-based guidelines and recommendations from reputable sources such as your pediatric health provider or a pediatric nutritionist. In Chapter 8, we'll walk through practical ways to find and confirm trustworthy resources that can support you in making informed decisions.

Family opinions often stem from personal experiences, cultural traditions, or beliefs that have been passed down through generations. While these perspectives should be respected, they may not always align with current scientific knowledge and guidelines. For instance, certain cultural practices or family preferences prioritize specific foods or eating patterns that may not provide a well-rounded and balanced diet.

To make informed decisions about children's food and eating patterns, it is essential to rely on evidence-based information.

Reputable sources can provide guidance on age-appropriate nutrition, portion sizes, food groups, and dietary recommendations specific to children. These sources take into account the nutritional needs and developmental stages of children, providing a foundation for making informed choices.

Pediatricians, in particular, can provide valuable guidance and address concerns related to a child's nutritional needs. They consider factors such as growth, allergies, and individual health conditions when making recommendations. By consulting with a healthcare professional, parents can receive personalized advice tailored to their child's specific needs.

Children's food preferences and eating behaviors can vary widely. While family members may have their own opinions about what a child should or should not eat, it's crucial to foster a positive and supportive eating environment. Pressuring children to eat specific foods or imposing strict dietary restrictions can lead to negative associations with food and potentially contribute to disordered eating patterns or nutritional deficiencies.

By combining the wisdom passed down through generations with evidence-based knowledge, parents can strike a balance that respects family values while prioritizing their child's nutritional needs. Open communication, respect for individual preferences, and a focus on health and well-being can help navigate the complexities of family opinions while ensuring the child receives a nourishing and balanced diet.

Here are some common topics where family members and friends often share their experiences and advice:

- **Breastfeeding-related changes:** If your baby is exclusively breastfed, family members may offer advice related to your diet. Some may suggest avoiding certain foods that are believed to cause digestive issues in the baby, such as spicy foods or ones that may "increase gas." While it's okay to make small changes in your diet in order to determine whether a food affects your infant's behavior, don't eliminate entire food groups unless you speak with a healthcare professional. It's vital for you to maintain a balanced and nutritious diet containing all food groups unless otherwise advised by a healthcare professional.

- **Formula-related changes:** If your baby is formula-fed, suggestions may include switching to a different formula brand or type. Some family members might believe that a specific formula can alleviate digestive issues or constipation. Consult with a healthcare professional before making any changes to your baby's formula. Generally, it is advisable to pick one formula and stick with it unless your healthcare provider recommends switching.

- **Introduction of solid foods:** Dozens of questions tend to arise when your baby starts solids. Should you make your own versus buy? What foods should you start with? Should you use organic versus non-organic? We have seen many parents with significant anxiety over all of these questions related to solid foods. It is important to know that there is not one absolute right or wrong way to start solids! As mentioned in Chapter 5, the introduction of solids should be done in consultation with a healthcare professional, following appropriate guidelines and considering the baby's developmental readiness. We urge families to be flexible when starting solids and know that there are many right ways to introduce solid foods!

- **Introducing rice cereal:** Family members may suggest adding rice cereal to your baby's bottle or starting solid foods earlier than recommended by the pediatrician. This is often based on the belief that the thicker consistency of the formula combined with rice cereal will help babies sleep better and for longer periods of time. Some also believe that the thicker formula can help reduce spitting up. However, introducing solids too early can have negative effects on a baby's digestive system (such as constipation and increased weight gain) and should only be done following the guidance of a healthcare professional. Generally, adding cereal to a bottle is not recommended.

- **Over-the-counter, herbal, or home remedies:** We recommend asking your pediatrician or healthcare provider before giving your baby any over the counter remedy-even if it is "natural." While some over-the-counter products are safe for infants, many are not recommended at all.

Gripe water is a popular example of a remedy for an irritable baby that is safe to try; just be sure to follow all recommended dosing guidelines. Gas drops (such as simethicone) are also commonly used. If your baby seems to have gas at the same time every day, you may give the medicine about thirty minutes before their "gassy" time. Some parents describe this as a miracle medicine, while others don't think it helps at all. If it doesn't provide any relief, then discontinue use.

Sometimes family members might propose using herbal teas, natural remedies, or over-the-counter medications to address changes in bowel movements, help with upper respiratory infections, or alleviate other symptoms. Please exercise caution, as some herbs or remedies may not be suitable for infants and can have potential side effects. Teas should never replace breast milk or formula because your infant always needs the nutrients and calories. And never give honey to any infant under the age of one! Talk to your pediatric health provider during your baby's well-child visits about any specific questions.

What to Expect—General Guidelines

Understanding normal variations in eating patterns and bowel movements in children is crucial for parents. While every child is unique, certain guidelines can help determine when a mother should be concerned and seek medical advice. These guidelines may vary depending on the age of the child. The following is a general overview.

Eating Patterns

In the early months, newborns have varying feeding patterns. Breastfed babies typically feed more frequently, while formula-fed babies may have longer intervals between feedings. As long as your baby is gaining weight, producing a sufficient number of wet diapers, and appears content after feedings, their eating patterns are likely normal. Seek medical advice if there are concerns about weight gain or signs of dehydration.

Poop Happens

When I worked as a pediatric nurse practitioner in gastroenterology and nutrition, parents often commented they never thought they would talk about poop so much! When I became a parent, our daily "How was your day, honey?" conversations inevitably included "How is the baby's poop?" Below are some tips on expected bowel movements and some information about advice you may receive from others. Approach these recommendations with caution and consult with a healthcare professional for accurate guidance.

Newborns typically have frequent bowel movements. Most often newborns will have stool several times per day; however, occasionally infants may go several days between bowel movements. Breastfed babies often have yellowish, seedy stools, while formula-fed babies may have firmer or pasty, tan-colored stools. As infants' guts are colonized with normal bacteria, their stools will start to smell. Generally, variations in consistency and frequency of stools are acceptable as long as feedings are not affected and your baby is otherwise acting normally. In some cases of constipation, giving your infant an ounce or two of prune juice can help soften the stool, but we recommend discussing this first with your pediatric provider. If your baby consistently experiences hard or pellet-like stools, displays concerning symptoms such as blood in the stool, aren't feeding well, seem uncomfortable, have a distended belly, or are acting lethargic, immediate medical advice should be sought.

In situations where the baby's bowel movements are causing distress or discomfort, healthcare professionals can evaluate potential causes such as food allergies, digestive issues, or infections. They can offer appropriate recommendations, such as dietary adjustments, probiotics, or further diagnostic tests if necessary.

Happy Spitters

Infants often experience a phase when they are referred to as "happy spitters." This term describes babies who spit up frequently but do not exhibit discomfort or distress associated with gastroesophageal reflux disease (GERD). For these infants, spitting up is a normal occurrence resulting from an underdeveloped lower esophageal sphincter. This muscle keeps stomach contents from rising up the esophagus. As they grow and mature, this muscle strengthens, typically resolving the issue. Happy spitters generally maintain a good appetite, gain weight appropriately, and exhibit cheerful and contented demeanors. Their spitting up is often painless and does not cause irritation or harm. It's a common part of infant development. In fact, happy spitting affects more than half of all babies! When our youngest was at home with his nanny, she knew she had to bring an extra set of clothes. When she washed his clothes, she threw her clothes in the washer as well! Despite the mess and many soiled clothes, he was quite content. Here are some tips to help.

- **Change the feeding position:** Altering the baby's feeding position, such as keeping them upright or at an inclined angle during and after feedings may help reduce the likelihood of spitting up by keeping the breast milk or formula from flowing back up easily.

- **Burp your baby more frequently:** Burping more often during and after feedings is a common suggestion to release any trapped air that could contribute to spitting up. You may want to try different burping techniques, such as gentle patting or holding the baby in an upright position while supporting their chin and back.

- **Adjusting the feeding schedule:** Feeding your baby smaller amounts more frequently can help. This approach aims to prevent your baby from taking in too much breast milk or formula at once, which could contribute to excessive spitting up.

- **Try different feeding techniques:** Using a slower flow nipple on the bottle or adjusting the breastfeeding latch to regulate the flow of milk may also lead to less spitting up. This can help prevent your baby from gulping down milk too quickly, potentially reducing the likelihood of spitting up.

When to Be Concerned

Every baby is unique, and what works for one may not work for another. While family recommendations can be valuable, it's crucial to prioritize evidence-based guidance from healthcare professionals such as your child's pediatrician, advanced practice provider, or nurse. While normal variations exist, there are certain red flags that indicate a need for medical attention regardless of age:

- Significant changes in eating habits, such as sudden refusal of all foods, persistent difficulty swallowing, or unexplained weight loss

- Projectile vomiting—more forceful than normal spit-ups, can even go across a room

- Persistent vomiting, especially if accompanied by fever, lethargy, or abdominal pain

- Vomiting that has blood in it, looks dark or has specks that mimic coffee grounds, or vomit that is bright yellow or green
- Severe or chronic constipation, particularly if it causes discomfort, bleeding, or impacts your baby's daily functioning
- Persistent diarrhea, especially if accompanied by dehydration, fever, blood in the stool, or other concerning symptoms
- Blood in the stool or dark, tarry stools
- Intolerances or allergic reactions to specific foods, such as severe allergic reactions (anaphylaxis), which may have symptoms such as hives, facial swelling, or difficulty breathing
- Failure to thrive, characterized by inadequate weight gain or growth compared to peers

Your pediatric healthcare provider will be monitoring your baby's growth at each well-child visit. Keeping these visits helps to ensure any signs of inadequate growth are recognized early.

Recognizing signs of dehydration in infants is also crucial, as they are more vulnerable to its effects. Here's a list of common signs and symptoms to watch for:

- **Dry mouth and tongue:** Your baby's mouth and tongue appear drier than usual.
- **No tears when crying:** An absence of tears when crying is a significant indicator.
- **Sunken soft spot on the head:** The soft spot (fontanelle) on the top of your baby's head may appear sunken.
- **Sunken eyes:** The eyes may look sunken or have dark circles around them.
- **Less-frequent urination:** Fewer wet diapers than usual (less than four to six wet diapers in twenty-four hours is a common benchmark).

- **Dark-yellow urine:** The urine may be darker and more concentrated than normal.

- **Lethargy or irritability:** Your baby may be unusually sleepy, less active, or more irritable than usual.

- **Cool and discolored hands and feet:** Your baby's hands and feet may feel cool to the touch and may look bluish or purple.

- **Poor skin elasticity:** When your baby's skin is gently pinched, it may not spring back as quickly as normal.

- **Rapid breathing or heart rate:** Your infant may breathe more rapidly or have a faster heartbeat.

- **Low energy levels or drowsiness:** Your baby seems unusually sluggish or sleepy.

- **Decreased responsiveness:** Your baby may not respond as actively to stimuli or may seem less alert.

If you notice any of these signs in your infant, seek medical attention immediately. Your provider or an emergency room provider can evaluate your child's overall health, conduct any necessary tests, and provide appropriate guidance or treatment. Dehydration can progress quickly and can be serious, especially in young children.

Every child is different, and there is a wide range of what can be considered normal. Trusting your motherly intuition is valuable, and seeking medical advice when there are concerns is always encouraged. Healthcare professionals are best equipped to assess the child's specific situation, provide accurate information, and offer appropriate support and interventions if needed.

Trust Your Intuition with the Help of the Holy Spirit

Throughout motherhood, listening for and recognizing the voice of the Holy Spirit amid the myriad voices and advice of others is crucial. We are first called to seek Jesus and develop a relationship with Him. We pray for the Holy Spirit to come to enlighten our hearts and minds and to send us good counsel by way of trusted family, friends, and professionals. We then discern the best choice for our baby. This discernment comes from a combination of knowledge, prayerful meditation, counsel of others, and practical experience.

The Holy Spirit speaks in alignment with biblical truths, providing guidance that is not only wise but also loving and peaceful.

Trusting our intuition is elevated and enriched by the experience of discernment with the help of the Holy Spirit. This divine guidance transcends human instinct, offering a deeper, more reliable source of wisdom and confidence. As we navigate the complexities of our responsibilities as mothers, we are reminded to listen to our instincts, seek counsel, and to hand the decision over to God for His guidance and wisdom. In doing so, we find ourselves continually led back to the loving embrace of the Trinity, empowered to act with confidence and purpose.

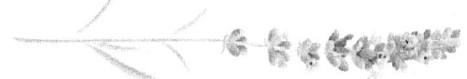

READ: *"Jesus said to her, 'Woman, why are you weeping? Whom are you looking for?' She thought it was the gardener and said to him, 'Sir, if you carried him away, tell me where you laid him, and I will take him.' Jesus said to her, 'Mary!' She turned and said to him in Hebrew, 'Rabbouni,' which means Teacher. . . . Mary of Magdala went and announced to the disciples, 'I have seen the Lord,' and what he told her.* (John 20:15–16, 18)

MEDITATE: Picture yourself searching for Christ with an open and humble heart. Feel the Spirit illuminating the path toward Christ. With confidence walk toward Him, step by step. Where is He leading you in the ordinary and sacred moments of your day?

PRAY: O, Holy Spirit, beloved of my soul, I adore you. Enlighten me, guide me, strengthen me, console me. Tell me what I should do; give me your orders. I promise to submit myself to all that you desire of me and to accept all that you permit to happen to me. Let me only know your will. Amen.[37]

LISTEN: "Goodness of God" by Bethel Music

RESOLVE: Write in your journal an example of the Holy Spirit encouraging, consoling, or guiding you.

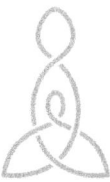

---

37   Cardinal Désiré-Joseph Mercier, "Prayer to the Holy Spirit," *Catholic Online*, accessed June 9, 2025, https://www.catholic.org/prayers/prayer.php?p=1404.

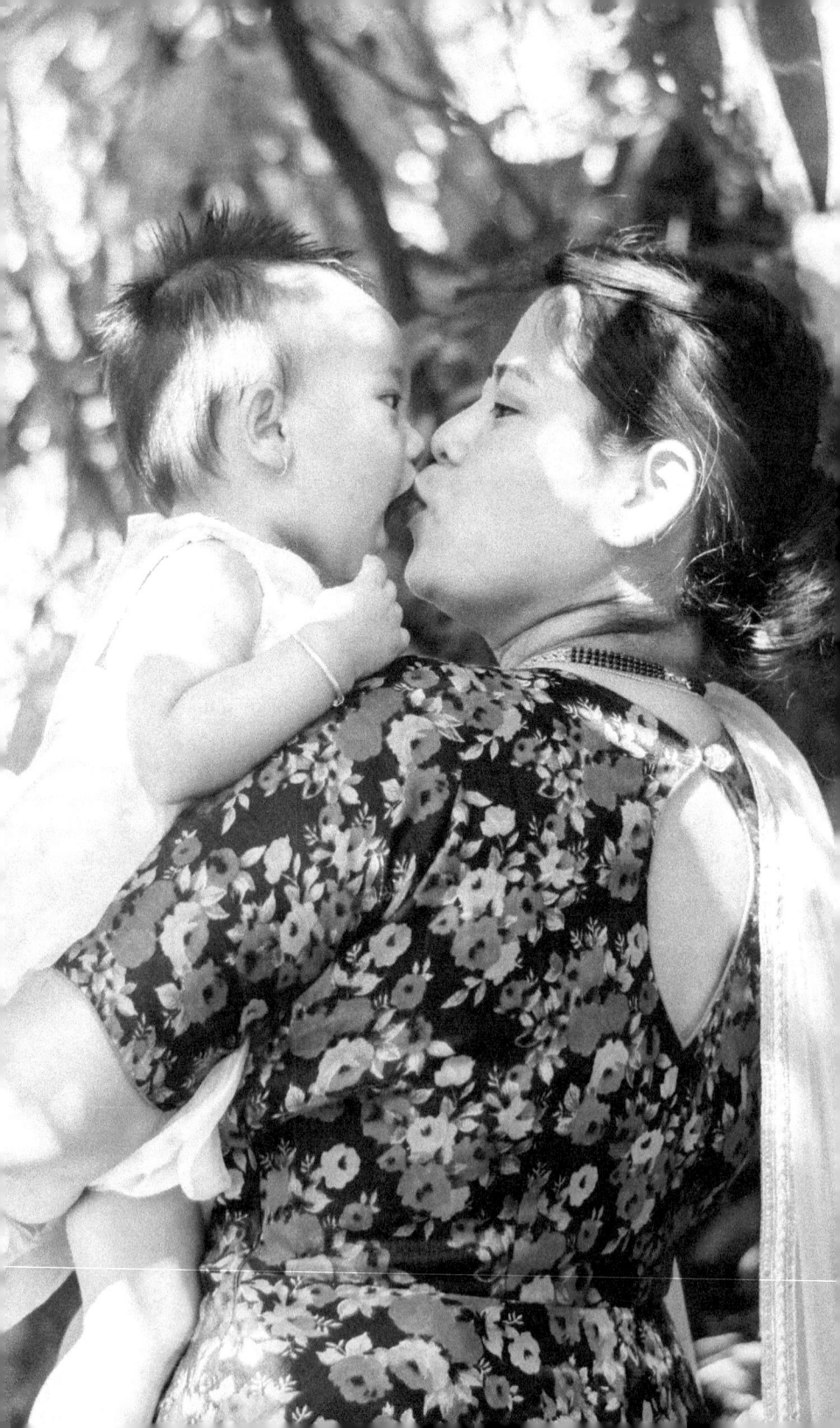

CHAPTER 7

You Are Beautiful
and Beloved!

"Jesus answered and said to her, 'If you knew the gift of God and who is saying to you, "Give me a drink," you would have asked him and he would have given you living water.'"

—John 4:10

During my freshman year of high school, I went to Mount Carmel Academy, an all-girls Catholic school in New Orleans. During every student assembly, the principal, a nun, would have all one thousand students stand and repeat after her: "I am beautiful, I am beautiful, I am beautiful!" She reminded us that our beauty comes from being a daughter of God, and He made us in His image and likeness. The Holy Spirit guides us to seek Jesus because He is waiting for us. Jesus reminds us of our inherent beauty not because of what we look like but because of who we are. Jesus is always waiting for us with open arms. He wants to meet us and fill us with the reminder of our beauty in Him and His living water of love. He is a true gentleman and will not force a relationship with us. He wants us to know and embrace the truth that He sees us for the beautiful person God created us to be.

You Are Seen and Loved

In Chapter 4 of John's Gospel, there is a powerful account of Jesus encountering a Samaritan woman at a well. The depth of Jesus' compassion and understanding is revealed by his desire to truly see her for the beautiful daughter of God that she was created to be. Despite the social and cultural barriers that separated them, Jesus saw the woman for who she truly was, engaging with her in a way that shattered the norms of his time. Even knowing her present living situation and past choices, he loved her and wanted to gift her with his living water. This story is another testimony to the dignity of women. He sees us in our struggles as mothers and wants to tell us that we are beautiful; he wants to give us his living water.

During Jesus' time, there existed a deep divide between Jews and Samaritans. This division was not only ethnic and cultural but also religious, as they had different beliefs and practices. The animosity between these two groups was such that Jews often avoided any contact or association with Samaritans. However, Jesus (a Jew), in his divine wisdom and love, chose to engage with this woman (a Samaritan). By breaking through the societal barriers and reaching out to her, he showed us that he calls everyone to his living water of love, truth, and beauty. He looks beyond our blemishes and sees our hearts. He wants to give us living water to quench our thirst and fill us with his love!

As Jesus approached the well, he asked the woman for a drink, initiating a conversation that would transform her life. This simple act of asking for water went against the norms of the time, as Jews were not expected to request anything from Samaritans. Jesus' desire to connect with her as a fellow human being surpassed cultural and religious boundaries.

Moreover, Jesus displayed an extraordinary ability to see into the depths of the woman's heart. In their conversation, Jesus revealed to the woman her past and present struggles, including her failed marriages and her longing for fulfillment. He acknowledged her pain and her search for love and acceptance, ultimately revealing himself as the source of living water that could quench her spiritual thirst.

"But whoever drinks the water I shall give will never thirst; the water I shall give will become in him a spring of water welling up to eternal life."

—John 4:14

When considering this story in the context of motherhood, we can think of the various challenges and struggles we face. The expectations, pressures, and judgments can weigh heavily on us, often leaving us feeling overwhelmed or inadequate. But just as Jesus saw the Samaritan woman and engaged with her on a personal level, He does the same for us. He shows us God's desire for a personal relationship with each of us, acknowledging our unique journey and struggles. He wants to give us living water so we can overflow with His love, truth, and grace.

While we look for beauty on the outside based on appearance, social status, employment, or financial means, Jesus looks beyond the surface. He dives deep into the well of our hearts, wishing to quench our thirst and fulfill our need for love. He sees the beauty and worth in each of us and calls us to worship Him in "spirit and truth" with sincerity and authenticity.

"God is Spirit, and those who worship him must worship in Spirit and truth."

—John 4:24

God wants us to care for our bodies because we were created in His image, and we are His temples. He also wants us to know that our outward appearance does not define who we are. He wants to meet us where we are, truly look at us, and then celebrate the joyful gift of His living water. As we take care of both ourselves and our babies, let us remember that true beauty comes from our loving Redeemer.

Mom's Skin Postpartum

After the miraculous journey of pregnancy and childbirth, women emerge as even more beautiful beings, bearing the marks of their transformative experience. As a new mom, I was self-conscious about the changes to my body, particularly in regard to my skin. Then someone told me that scars are a way for the light of Jesus to shine through me. These reminders can be viewed as a testament of our strength and resilience. From stretch marks to pigmentation variations, these physical alterations tell a unique story of creation and nurturing.

Each mark represents the remarkable growth of new life within and the sacrifices made to bring forth a new generation. We can choose to embrace these changes as symbols of their love, power, and motherhood. The lines etched on our bodies can serve as a reminder of the incredible capacity of our bodies.

In the end, a woman's beauty lies not in the absence of change, but in her ability to embrace and celebrate every transformation. In this way the beauty of strength, resilience, and the unbreakable bond between you and Jesus shines forth.

The following is some practical advice about how to care for your new beauty marks.

EPISIOTOMY

When I gave birth to my first son, my physician had to perform an episiotomy and the delivery did the rest, leaving me with a third-degree tear. When the bottle of pain medicine was empty and I was still at a pain level of six out of ten, I knew something was wrong. After seeing the doctor, I was instructed to do sitz baths (a warm, shallow bath) four times daily to encourage healing; if that didn't do the trick, surgery might be required.

Nobody talks about the challenges of balancing postpartum constipation, pain medicine, hemorrhoids from delivery and caring for an episiotomy. The struggle was real! It was a lot to deal with on top of learning how to breastfeed and care for a newborn.

Here are some essential tips to provide proper care for your skin to optimize healing and minimize discomfort after undergoing an often necessary but always uncomfortable episiotomy:

- **Keep the area clean:** A peri-bottle is your friend! If you need to wipe the area, do so with a wet soft cloth using a patting motion. Take sitz baths. Ask your healthcare provider if you can add anything to the plain water or whether there are restrictions depending on the type of delivery and/or stitches you may have. When done, pat dry. Talk to your provider before applying ointments or creams as each one works in a unique way.

- **Prevent constipation:** Talk to your healthcare provider about a stool softener because constipation will cause unnecessary discomfort and potentially worsen any skin tears. Drink plenty of water and supplement dietary fiber with psyllium fiber powder. Put your feet on a one-foot tall stool or bench (such as a squatty potty) when having a bowel movement. This will optimize body alignment, prevent straining, and maximize stool evacuation from your bowel.

- **Manage pain and discomfort:** Use over-the-counter pain relievers or prescribed medications as directed by your doctor to alleviate pain and reduce swelling. Applying a cold pack wrapped in a thin cloth can also provide relief. Do not apply any ice directly to your skin; this can cause burning.

- **Practice good hygiene:** Change sanitary pads frequently because any moistness on your skin can cause further breakdown. Opt for pads that are breathable and non-irritating. Avoid tampons until your healthcare provider gives you the green light.

- **Promote air circulation:** Sit on a donut pillow or soft egg foam. Wear loose-fitting cotton underwear to allow air circulation and minimize friction on the incision area.

- **Stay hydrated and eat well:** A healthy diet rich in protein, fiber, and nutrients and drinking plenty of water can aid in the healing process. Keep your snack baskets full of high fiber, high protein snacks. Greek yogurt is a great source of protein and provides probiotics. Talk to your healthcare provider before starting a daily probiotic supplement.

- **Balance movement with taking it easy:** Avoid strenuous activities, heavy lifting, and prolonged sitting to prevent added pressure on the incision area. Gentle walking helps ensure your bowels are moving and is excellent for keeping your muscles active.

Remember, every woman's healing process is unique. If you have concerns or experience unusual symptoms, always consult with your healthcare provider for personalized guidance and support.

BREAST ENGORGEMENT

As your body transforms to enable you to feed your baby, breast engorgement can cause skin to become tight, swollen, and sensitive, creating discomfort and potentially causing nipple cracking or irritation. Here are some tips to care for your skin during this bumpy ride:

- **Warm compresses:** Apply a warm compress or take a warm shower before nursing or pumping to help soften the breasts and ease milk flow.

- **Cold packs:** Cold compresses or chilled cabbage leaves can provide significant relief from breast engorgement discomfort between feedings. Apply them for fifteen to twenty minutes at a time after nursing (rather than right before) to minimize any potential impact on milk supply while still benefiting from the anti-inflammatory effects. If you use ice, be sure to protect your skin with a thin cloth so as not to cause frostbite or cold injury. I used circular nursing pads from the freezer to help the engorgement. I wore a thin camisole, then cold packs, followed by my nursing bra and a T-shirt.

- **Proper support:** Invest in a well-fitting, supportive bra that doesn't constrict or dig into your skin. It is well worth the money. You want your breasts to have good blood and lymphatic circulation for optimal breastfeeding and to prevent mastitis.

- **Hydration and nutrition:** Stay hydrated and maintain a healthy diet to support milk production and overall skin health.

- **Gentle massage:** Use gentle circular motions and apply a mild moisturizer to soothe tightness and promote circulation.

- **Nurse or pump frequently:** Regularly emptying your breasts helps prevent further engorgement and keeps your milk supply in check.

- **Seek help if needed:** If engorgement persists or becomes painful, consult a lactation consultant or healthcare professional for further guidance and support. You're not alone in this journey!

ACNE

Postpartum acne can be caused by various factors, including hormonal fluctuations, stress, and changes in your skincare routine. After giving birth, hormone levels, particularly estrogen and progesterone, undergo significant shifts, which can trigger increased oil production and clogged pores, leading to acne breakouts. The stress associated with adjusting to motherhood, sleep deprivation, and lifestyle changes can also contribute to acne flare-ups. Additionally, using certain favorite products may no longer suit your post-pregnancy skin. Each woman's experience is unique, and consulting with a healthcare professional or dermatologist can provide personalized insight and guidance to manage postpartum acne effectively.

Post-pregnancy acne can be frustrating. Here's a quick guide to tackle those pesky pimples:

- **Cleanse gently:** Use a mild, non-comedogenic cleanser to cleanse your face twice a day. Avoid harsh scrubbing or over-cleansing. Consider Vanicream or Cetaphil moisturizing face washes for a simple routine until the hormones settle down.

- **Moisturize wisely:** Choose an oil-free, non-greasy moisturizer to hydrate your skin without clogging pores. Vanicream and Cetaphil come highly recommended by dermatologists.

- **Spot treat:** Use over-the-counter acne treatments with ingredients like benzoyl peroxide or salicylic acid to target individual breakouts.[38] Resist the temptation to pick or squeeze acne, as it can lead to scarring and further inflammation.

- **Live a healthy lifestyle:** Maintain a balanced diet, stay hydrated, and get regular exercise to support overall skin health.

---

38   S. Ly, K. Kamal, P. Manjaly, S.J. Barbieri, and A. Mostaghimi, "Treatment of Acne Vulgaris During Pregnancy and Lactation: A Narrative Review," *Dermatology and Therapy (Heidelberg)*. 2023 Jan;13(1):115–130.

- **Seek professional help:** If acne persists or worsens, consult a dermatologist for personalized treatment options.

Remember, this too shall pass, and you'll soon be glowing with that new mom radiance!

C-SECTION SCAR

Caring for a C-section scar is crucial for proper healing and minimizing discomfort. Here are some tips:

- **Keep it clean:** Gently clean the incision site with mild soap and warm water. Pat dry with a clean towel. Only apply prescribed ointments or dressings if directed by your healthcare provider; instructions should be listed on your hospital discharge paperwork.

- **Protect and support:** Consider wearing a supportive abdominal binder or underwear to provide gentle compression and reduce strain on the incision. If you choose to use some kind of compression, make sure it is not too tight as this can actually impede healing. Keep the remainder of your clothing loose to prevent rubbing against the scar and opt for loose-fitting, breathable garments.

- **Massage to prevent adhesions:** After about six to eight weeks, discuss with your healthcare provider whether you may gently massage the scar with a moisturizer. This can help prevent adhesions and promote circulation. Use the pads of your fingers and massage in all directions. I wish I had known this advice earlier! It took several years for my scar to loosen up.

- **Avoid sun exposure:** Protect the scar from direct sunlight as it may darken and become more noticeable.

- **Be patient:** C-section scars take time to fade and flatten. Give yourself ample rest and recovery time.

Remember, each person's healing journey is unique. If you have concerns or notice any unusual symptoms such as redness, increased pain, drainage, or fever, be sure to consult your healthcare provider immediately for personalized advice and support.

Baby's Skin

New babies often experience skin issues as their skin matures outside of your womb and changes without your hormones. An infant's skin is significantly different from adult skin, and it undergoes remarkable changes during the first twelve months of life. For example:

Infant skin is thinner and more delicate, making it susceptible to dryness, irritation, and sensitivity.

An infant's skin barrier is not fully developed, allowing substances to penetrate more easily. This makes them more vulnerable to chemicals, allergens, and infections.

- Infant skin has higher trans-epidermal water loss, making it more prone to dryness. Regular moisturizing with a fragrance-free moisturizer is essential to maintain hydration.

- Infants struggle to regulate their body temperature efficiently, so they are more susceptible to overheating or getting cold. For the first two to three months, clothing your baby in one more layer of clothing than what you are wearing is a practical tip.[39]

- Constant exposure to moisture, friction, and irritants in the diaper area can lead to diaper rash.

- Hormonal changes and exposure to new environments can cause baby acne, milia, or various rashes, including eczema and cradle cap.[40]

---

39   American Academy of Pediatrics, "Tips for Dressing Your Baby," *HealthyChildren.org*. accessed April 28, 2025, https://www.healthychildren.org/English/ages-stages/baby/diapers-clothing/Pages/Dressing-Your-Newborn.aspx.

40   "Newborn Skin 101," *Hopkins Medicine*, accessed April 28, 2025, https://www.hopkinsmedicine.org/health/wellness-and-prevention/newborn-skin-101.

Understanding these differences helps parents take appropriate care of their baby's skin by using gentle (fragrance-free) cleansers, moisturizers, and avoiding harsh chemicals or irritants. Regular monitoring and seeking medical advice for persistent or concerning skin conditions is crucial during the first year of a baby's life.

BATHING

Bathing is an essential part of caring for your baby. Here are important guidelines to follow:

- **Bathing frequency:** For the first one to two weeks of life, babies should only receive sponge baths. Once their umbilical cord stump falls off and the area heals, you may begin to give your child a more typical bath. Generally, most babies only need bathing once every two to three days for the first year of life.[41]

- **Water temperature:** Ensuring the water temperature is just right can prevent burns but also can help prevent skin from drying out. Water should feel warm to the touch and not hot. The American Academy of Pediatrics recommends that hot water heaters in homes with children be set to no more than 120 degrees Fahrenheit to avoid the risk of scalding injuries.[42]

- **Gentle cleansing:** Use a mild, fragrance-free cleanser specifically formulated for bath time. Use soap sparingly and be gentle when washing their skin. Infant skin does not need harsh scrubbing. Once your infant is a little older and more interactive, it's okay to let them have some quick playtime in the bath if they are having fun. However, remember that the longer they are in the bath, the more their skin may dry out.

41 American Academy of Pediatrics, "Bathing Your Newborn," *HealthyChildren.org*, accessed April 28, 2025, https://www.healthychildren.org/English/ages-stages/baby/bathing-skin-care/Pages/Bathing-Your-Newborn.aspx.

42 American Academy of Pediatrics, "Bathing Your Newborn."

- **Bathing the private areas:** The last step of the bath should be to gently cleanse the diaper area. If your son's penis is circumcised, follow the instructions provided by the hospital. If your son's penis is not circumcised, during bath time simply wash the genitals gently with water and soap. You should not pull back the foreskin of an infant since this can lead to scarring, pain, and sometimes even bleeding. As your child grows, the foreskin will gradually separate from the glans.[43]

- **After the bath:** Have a towel nearby so you can wrap your baby from head to toe once bathing is complete. Gently pat your baby dry following bath time, being sure to dry creases and folds. After they are dry, apply a fragrance-free moisturizer to keep your baby's skin hydrated. Choose products that are hypoallergenic without harsh chemicals.

DIAPER CARE

Proper diaper care is essential for your baby's comfort and overall well-being. Here are some tips to keep in mind:

- **Diaper-changing routine:** Change diapers frequently to prevent prolonged exposure to moisture and reduce the risk of diaper rash. Clean the diaper area with gentle wipes or a damp cloth, wiping from front to back. If the skin is not soiled, you can air dry. This is a great time to do a minute or two of tummy time! Roll your baby over and put their hands by their shoulders. Stay standing with them, talking to them while they get a miniature exercise workout.

- **Diaper choice matters:** Choose diapers that are gentle on the skin, breathable, and absorbent. Consider using diapers

---

43   American Academy of Pediatrics, "Care for an Uncircumcised Penis," *HealthyChildren.org*, accessed April 28, 2025, https://www.healthychildren.org/English/ages-stages/baby/bathing-skin-care/Pages/Care-for-an-Uncircumcised-Penis.aspx.

free from chlorine, fragrances, and harsh chemicals. You may have to experiment with a few diaper brands before finding the right fit for your baby. In recent years, cloth diapers have become more popular again. Some moms choose these diapers for environmental reasons, cost, and versatility. As with many parental decisions, there are advantages and disadvantages to choosing cloth diapers. Be flexible and take the time to explore what is best for your family and personal situation.

- **Diaper-free time:** Give your baby some diaper-free time to allow their skin to breathe and reduce the likelihood of diaper rash. Place a waterproof mat or towel underneath them for easy cleanup.

- **Diaper rash prevention:** Use a barrier cream or ointment with each diaper change to protect your baby's skin from moisture and friction. Avoid products containing potential irritants such as fragrance or dyes. If your baby does develop diaper rash, treating it with a diaper ointment containing a high percentage of zinc oxide is a good choice. I often told patients to apply the diaper ointment in a thick layer so the skin was not even visible!

- **Signs of irritation:** Regularly inspect your baby's skin for any redness, rashes, or signs of discomfort. Consult a healthcare professional if you notice persistent or severe diaper rash.

Each baby's skin is unique, and it's important to choose products and practices that suit their individual needs. Keeping their skin clean, moisturized, and dry, along with diligent diaper care, helps promote a healthy and happy baby.

CRADLE CAP

Cradle cap is a common skin condition that appears as thick, crusty, or scaly patches on a baby's scalp. It may also occur on the eyebrows, eyelids, or behind the ears. It is usually harmless and doesn't cause discomfort to the baby. Here are some recommendations for caring for cradle cap based on guidance from the American Academy of Pediatrics (AAP):

- **Gentle cleansing:** Use a mild baby shampoo and gently massage the scalp to loosen the scales. Avoid picking or scratching, as this can lead to skin irritation.

- **Soft brushing:** After shampooing, use a soft brush or a clean, soft cloth to gently remove the loosened scales. Be gentle to avoid causing any discomfort or injury to the baby's delicate skin.

- **Baby oil:** Apply a small amount of baby oil or petroleum jelly to the affected areas to help soften and moisturize the scales. Leave it on for a short period before gently washing it off during the next bath.

- **Consult your pediatrician:** If cradle cap persists, becomes severe, or spreads to other areas of the body, consult your pediatrician. They may recommend medicated shampoos, creams, or ointments to manage the condition.

Cradle cap usually resolves on its own over time. With gentle care and patience, you can effectively manage it while ensuring the well-being of your baby's scalp and skin.[44]

INFANT ACNE

Identifying and treating infant acne requires understanding its characteristics and taking gentle care of your baby's delicate skin. Infant acne typically appears as small red bumps or whiteheads on the face, especially the cheeks and forehead. Unlike adult acne, it

---

44   American Academy of Pediatrics, "Cradle Cap," *HealthyChildren.org*, accessed April 28, 2025. https://www.healthychildren.org/English/ages-stages/baby/bathing-skin-care/Pages/Cradle-Cap.aspx.

is not caused by clogged pores or excess oil production. Most cases of infant acne resolve on their own without intervention. To treat it, avoid applying any creams or lotions, as they can worsen the condition. Instead, gently cleanse the affected area with warm water and a mild baby cleanser. Pat dry and let the skin breathe, avoiding any harsh rubbing or scrubbing. If you have concerns or if the acne persists or worsens, consult your pediatrician for further guidance and reassurance.

UNDERSTANDING THAT MARBLED LOOK

When I was growing up in the 1990s, Hypercolor shirts were a popular fashion trend in the United States. The pigments in the fabric reacted to hot temperatures, causing the shirt to shift hues. At times, your baby's skin may resemble those totally awesome shirts from my childhood! This skin condition is sometimes referred to as "mottled skin."

Mottled skin in newborns refers to a blotchy or marbled appearance of the skin, characterized by areas of different colors, often seen as patches of pale or reddish-blue skin. This phenomenon is usually normal and commonly occurs due to the immaturity of the baby's circulatory system. Mottling can be more noticeable when your baby is cold, as blood vessels constrict, or when they are warm, as blood vessels dilate. These changes in baby skin appearance are typically harmless and resolve on their own as the baby's circulatory system matures.

However, if mottling is accompanied by other worrisome symptoms like difficulty breathing, lethargy, poor feeding, or cyanosis (blue color to lips, skin, and nailbeds), seek medical attention promptly.

Monitoring your baby's overall well-being, ensuring they are appropriately dressed for the temperature, and seeking medical advice when necessary are key factors in promoting the health and comfort of your little one's skin.

ALWAYS HAVE AN EXTRA SET OF CLOTHES!

Having an extra set of clothes on hand for you and your baby at all times is an easy way to promote skin health. Accidents happen, and damp or soiled clothes can lead to irritation and discomfort, especially for delicate baby skin. By having spare clothing on hand, you can quickly change your baby's clothes, ensuring they stay clean and dry. Additionally, if you or your baby experience any spills or leaks, changing into fresh clothes helps maintain proper hygiene and prevents skin irritation. I recommend having a packed bag of extras that stays in your car. My oldest had a massive blowout at church, and having an extra nursing bra and shirt to change into saved the day! It's a simple yet effective way to prioritize the well-being of both Mom and baby.

In Summary

The story of the woman at the well shows us that Jesus sees beyond physical appearance to our true identity as beloved daughters of God. This is true especially during the postpartum period, when our bodies show the marks of bringing new life into the world. Just as Jesus offered living water to the Samaritan woman, He offers us the grace to see our changing bodies through His eyes.

Sweet sister, God wants to remind you that your body is a temple of the Holy Spirit. Just as you gently care for your baby's delicate skin, He invites you to care for your own postpartum body with the same tenderness—without guilt or shame. These small, intentional acts of care are not vain; they are beautiful expressions of motherhood that reflect His love and design. True beauty flows from knowing we are deeply loved by God. Like the Samaritan woman at the well, our worth isn't found in appearances or what we have done. Instead our beauty and worth is found in who we are in Him. So take a deep breath, care for yourself as you do your little one, and trust that Jesus sees every moment as sacred.

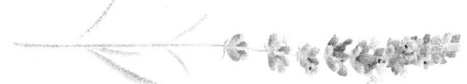

READ: *"If you knew the gift of God, and who it is that asks you for a drink, you would have asked him and he would have given you living water."* (John 4:10)

MEDITATE: Envision Jesus waiting for you to quench your thirst and remind you that you are a beautiful daughter of God.

PRAY: Lord, give me the strength to meet you at the well, to accept the truth of my beauty and an open heart to receive your living water.

LISTEN: "Beautiful" by Mercy Me

RESOLVE

1. Write in your journal how Jesus met you where you needed Him most.
2. Pack a bag with an extra set of clothes, diapers, wipes, and burp cloth—and remember to put it in the car!

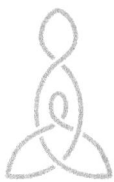

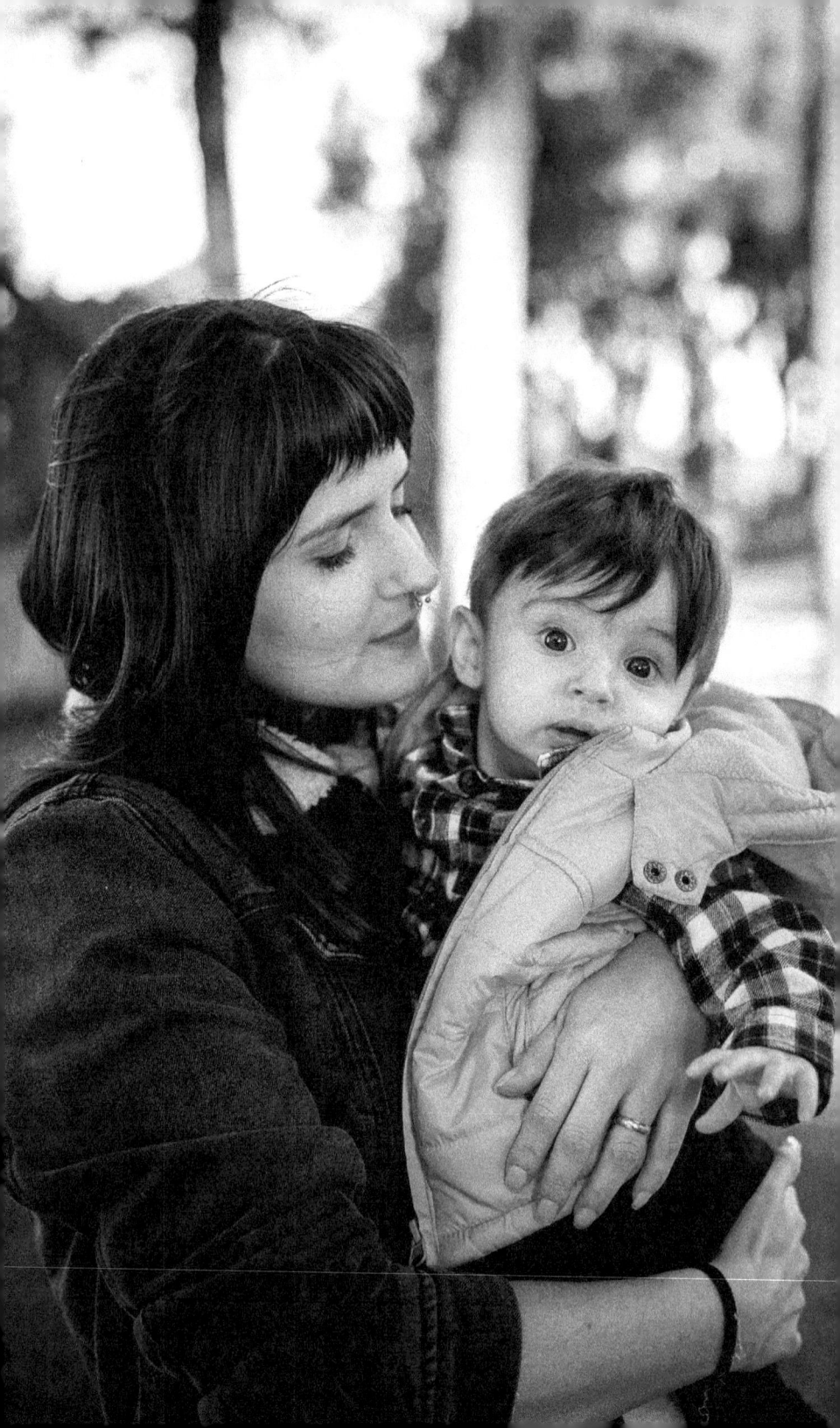

CHAPTER 8

Where to Get Help

"Indeed, the word of God is living and effective,
sharper than any two-edged sword, penetrating even
between soul and spirit, joints and marrow, and able to
discern reflections and thoughts of the Heart."

—Hebrews 4:12

This past summer, I was given my grandmother's Bible. The pocket-sized King James Bible with the gilded edges and red leather cover now opens easily given the many years of use. When I saw my grandmother's handwritten notes and underlined verses, I could hear her wit and her kind but strong voice. She was the wife of an Air Force pilot during World War II, often raising four children by herself in a foreign country. From conversations with her before she passed, I know God's Word and the truth of His love written throughout the Bible were sources of strength for her.

In today's age, we are bombarded with information and messages more than at any other time in human history. Technology continues to progress at lightning speed and artificial intelligence (AI) now offers many promises of quickly obtaining desired information. However, if the information feeding the algorithms is not credible, the resulting answers are suspect. AI combined with all the information on social media makes true knowledge hard to find and wisdom difficult to obtain. As believers in Christ, we are assured that we are not alone. God, in His almighty wisdom and love for us, ensured we were given the power of His Word in the Bible. Remember, the Bible is just as applicable for us today as it was for those living when it was written.

History tells of women who led lives that exemplified how the truths of the Bible are our steady source of truth and comfort today and always.

St. Margaret

St. Margaret of Scotland was a deeply devout Christian, wife, mother, and queen. Her faith profoundly influenced her rule and significantly impacted religious and cultural life in her kingdom. Born around 1045 into English royalty, Margaret was exiled to Scotland following the Norman invasion of England. There, she married King Malcolm III and became Queen of Scotland.

St. Margaret was most notable for her dedication to the Bible. Her commitment to Scripture was unusual for her time, especially for a woman. She led by example as a unique royal who read the Bible regularly and encouraged others to do the same. She also made sure her eight children were well-versed in the Bible. This upbringing had a lasting impact, as several of her children later became notable figures in religious and political history.

Her dedication to the Bible deeply informed her actions as queen. She used scriptural teachings as her guide, striving to rule justly and compassionately. Margaret was known for her charitable works, and she shared her riches with the poor. She was instrumental in founding churches and monasteries and in promoting the observance of Christian feasts and rituals. The small Bible that she carried, a gift from her husband, was beautifully adorned and decorated. Once, the Bible fell in the river but was thankfully retrieved! Amazingly, the Bible was not damaged and can still be viewed today. St. Margaret's legacy is a testament to the transformative power of the Bible in individual and societal life.

"Stand firm then, with the belt of truth buckled around your waist, with the breastplate of righteousness in place."

—Ephesians 6:14

St. Paul encouraged the early Christians to arm themselves with the truths of the Bible. This still rings true today. As mothers, we need the Bible's love letters to us from God to fill our daily lives. As we relive the stories, we can learn important lessons from the men and women who came before us. The teachings offer practical advice for the challenges of daily life and spiritual security and growth. The Bible narratives exemplify virtues such as kindness, compassion, resilience, and faith, sound reminders for us and qualities that we strive to instill in our children.

Prayer is another source of finding truth. We know that God sent His only Son to us so we may be forgiven and redeemed. In prayer, we are able to communicate with our Almighty Father, His Son, and the Holy Spirit—the ultimate sources of truth and power.

One of my favorite stories in the Bible is the widow that keeps asking the judge for justice (see Luke 18:1–8). Ultimately, he gives her what she is asking because of her persistence! God wants us to persist in prayer. He does hear us, and He answers according to His will.

Trustworthy Information and Your Spiritual Growth

The Bible and prayer serve as powerful resources for seeking help and finding solace in times of need. They offer guidance, encouragement, and a sense of connection to a higher power. Whether facing challenges, seeking guidance, or finding comfort, turning to the Bible and praying can provide strength and reassurance. Here, we explore the significance of the Bible and prayer as resources for help, drawing inspiration from impactful Bible verses.

Fill us with your love, O Lord, and we will sing for joy (Psalms 94:10). This verse reminds us that the Lord is our source of joy and strength. He wants us to live each day close to Him, allowing His love to infuse our hearts and be our source of joy. Knowing we are redeemed, loved, and chosen brings joy and strengthens us throughout the day.

Ask and it will be given to you; seek and you will find; knock and the door will be opened to you. For everyone who asks, receives; and the one who seeks, finds; and to the one who knocks, the door will be opened (Matthew 7:7–8). Jesus encourages us to seek God's help through prayer and assures us that our requests will be heard. This passage reminds us of the power of prayer as a means of communication with God and a way to seek guidance and assistance. We can approach God with confidence, knowing He will respond to our requests according to His divine wisdom.

Have no anxiety at all, but in everything, by prayer and petition, with thanksgiving, make your requests known to God. Then the peace of God that surpasses all understanding will guard your hearts and minds in Christ Jesus (Philippians 4:6–7). This verse is one of the best ones for us to turn to when we are anxious. The apostle Paul encourages and reminds us not to be consumed by anxiety but to bring our concerns and requests to God in prayer. We often need to be gently reminded of the importance of maintaining a thankful and prayerful attitude in all situations. God wants us to experience His peace, which surpasses human understanding. It's a peace that guards our hearts and minds.

They that hope in the Lord will renew their strength, they will soar on eagles' wings; they will run and not grow weary, walk and not grow faint (Isaiah 40:31). God is with us always. This is true in times of distress or weariness and in times of contentment and celebration. He wants us to soar and live the beautiful life He has planned for us. When we meditate on this verse, we can imagine ourselves strong and living a life that shines God's glory.

God has written a love letter filled with instructions for every season, emotion, and experience in our life. He wants to communicate His unending presence and love to us. He wants us to turn to Him, to get to know Him. Just like we want to soak up every beautiful inch of our sweet babies, God wants the same relationship with us. He knows that the more we know Him, the more grounded, confident, and joyful we will be in this life. These truths are only the beginning; we also have an amazing life in eternity waiting for us! Turn to the Bible to renew your strength, seek guidance, accept comfort, grow in hope, and offer praise! The Bible and prayer provide a foundation of faith, hope, and guidance for our spiritual health and a solid ground for living your life.

Reputable Resources

Just as we seek resources for our spiritual wellness through the Bible and direct communication with God in prayer, knowing where to go for trustworthy information for your child's health is important. Seeking professional help and counsel for practical solutions to whole health is a wise decision. While social media offers readily accessible health information, many self-proclaimed experts share advice without proper medical credentials or training.

When it comes to making decisions about our children's well-being, we want to rely on reputable sources of information. The choices we make for our children can have long-lasting effects on their health and development. Choosing and establishing a primary care medical home with a pediatrician, pediatric nurse practitioner, or family practice provider provides an environment for a trained professional to get to know you and your child. The primary care provider will help you ensure the well-child visits and all recommended needs for your child's well-being are accurately performed in a timely manner.

While recommendations from family and friends can be a great starting point in finding the right provider for your infant, take the time to do your own research. Each child and family is unique, so investing some time to explore your options can make a real difference in your child's healthcare journey. We have included some tips for selecting a pediatric provider for your family in Appendix 1.

FINDING SOURCES OF TRUSTWORTHY INFORMATION

In our journey of motherhood, seeking reliable information is crucial, but it's equally important to approach all sources with a discerning and thoughtful perspective. Organizations like the American Academy of Pediatrics (AAP) and major academic pediatric institutions continue to provide rigorously researched, evidence-based guidance grounded in clinical expertise. The U.S. Centers for Disease Control and Prevention (CDC) also produces valuable technical resources, such as developmental milestones and data reports, though some of its public-facing messaging has recently shifted in ways that have raised questions for many parents and clinicians. For that reason, drawing from a variety of trusted medical sources and discussing any uncertainties with your child's pediatrician can be especially helpful.

These trusted sources dedicate themselves to evaluating the best scientific evidence to support child health. However, medical knowledge is always evolving, recommendations can shift as new research emerges, and even respected institutions can be subtly influenced by broader cultural, economic, and political contexts. This doesn't diminish their value; instead it invites us to be thoughtful consumers of information. Approach these sources with both respect and critical thinking: Read widely, ask questions, consult multiple sources, discuss recommendations with your pediatrician, and always filter guidance through your own intuition and specific family circumstances. Your informed, loving judgment as a mother is an essential complement to professional medical advice.

WHEN MEDICAL ADVICE CHANGES: A SIGN OF PROGRESS

As a pediatrician and mother, I've witnessed multiple shifts in medical recommendations throughout my career. These changes do not mean previous advice was wrong. Instead, they reflect our growing understanding of children's health.

One example that illustrates this change relates to food allergies. For years, pediatricians recommended delaying the introduction of highly allergenic foods like peanuts until after a child's first birthday. This seemed logical at the time. Then came the groundbreaking LEAP (Learning Early About Peanut Allergy) study in 2015, which showed that early introduction of peanut products to high-risk infants dramatically reduced their chance of developing peanut allergies.[45] This evidence completely reversed our previous guidance! Now we recommend introducing peanut-containing foods as early as four to six months for most infants.

Similarly, infant sleep recommendations transformed dramatically in the 1990s. For generations, parents were advised to place babies on their stomachs to sleep, believing this reduced the risk of choking. When research revealed this position actually increased SIDS risk, the "Back to Sleep" campaign was launched. The simple change of placing babies on their backs to sleep has reduced SIDS deaths by more than 50 percent.[46]

These evolving recommendations are not signs of medical uncertainty but rather scientific progress in action. As physicians, we continually refine our advice as new evidence emerges. As parents, embracing these changes, even when they contradict what we did with our older children, means providing the best care based on our current understanding. When medical advice shifts, it is not a weakness in medicine but rather shows the commitment to following evidence toward better outcomes for our children.

---

45   G. Du Toit, G. Roberts, P.H. Sayre, et al, "Randomized Trial of Peanut Consumption in Infants at Risk for Peanut Allergy," *New England Journal of Medicine*, 2015 Feb 26;372(9):803–813.

46   "Data & Research: SIDS Deaths by Cause," Centers for Disease Control and Prevention, accessed March 13, 2025, https://www.cdc.gov/sudden-infant-death/data-research/data/sids-deaths-by-cause.html.

When evaluating sources, here are some specific details to consider:

- **Credibility:** Assess the reputation and expertise of the organization or author. Look for credentials, affiliations, and a history of publishing reliable information.

- **Timeliness:** Check when the information was last updated. Science and medical knowledge are constantly evolving, so it's essential to have access to the most recent research and recommendations that are based on evidence.

- **Consistency:** Verify that the information aligns with recommendations from other reputable sources. Consensus among multiple trusted sources adds weight to the information provided.

- **Transparency:** Reputable sources are transparent about their sources of funding and potential conflicts of interest. This transparency helps ensure the information is not influenced by biased agendas.

- **Accessibility:** Reliable sources provide clear and understandable information targeted to a diverse audience, including parents and caregivers.

When making decisions about your children's well-being, you can use these tips to help you discern which resources are trustworthy. Reputable sources provide objective and up-to-date information, whereas family opinions can be influenced by personal experiences, biases, and limited knowledge. The opinions of others may be a good starting place to inquire further about what is best, and it's possible that ultimately the opinion may be the best decision. However, you want to first thoughtfully consider the information, turn to trusted sources, prayerfully consider what is best for your child, and then make a loving decision to promote the health, safety, and optimal development of your child.

One resource we recommend is the AAP website for parents: **www.healthychildren.org**. It's easy to navigate and is organized in a user-friendly manner. This resource provides articles, medication dosing information for over-the-counter medicine such as ibuprofen, developmental milestones, and much more. The website is also available in Spanish.

The CDC website is another excellent resource with seemingly endless tools, videos, checklists, and articles. One favorite is the milestones page[47] that contains photos and videos to help parents and caregivers know what to expect as their baby grows. As with any resource, read for consistency across other trusted websites and assess if the most recent updates match credible authors and evidence based science.

Another resource that we recommend is **KidsHealth.org**, which offers healthcare information directed at both parents and children. The WebMD Parenting Section also offers helpful advice and education for parents. State health departments, well-known children's hospitals, and the Women, Infants, and Children (WIC) Nutrition Program websites are also places where you can find resources to assist you in parenting. This information is generally trusted and relied upon by healthcare professionals, policymakers, and parents alike.

The resources above provide comprehensive education on immunizations, including recommended schedules, safety information, and answers to frequently asked questions. Their guidance is grounded in extensive research and designed to protect children from vaccine-preventable diseases. Nutrition, sleep, healthy growth, and safety are other topics thoroughly presented. You can discuss the information with your baby's pediatric healthcare provider. Use the information to write questions before your

---

47   "Developmental Milestones," Centers for Disease Control and Prevention, accessed February 13, 2025, https://www.cdc.gov/ncbddd/actearly/milestones/index.html.

well-child visit to ensure you feel well-informed about your decisions for your child.

AAP SYMPTOM CHECKER

The American Academy of Pediatrics (AAP) provides a valuable symptom checker that can help you make informed decisions when you're unsure whether to take your child to the emergency department. This resource is available online at **https://www. healthychildren.org/English/tips-tools/Symptom-Checker/ Pages/default.aspx** and serves as a trusted guide, offering reliable information and recommendations based on pediatric expertise. It covers a wide range of symptoms and conditions, providing detailed explanations and guidance on when to seek emergency care, when to contact a healthcare provider, and when home care may be sufficient.

The AAP Symptom Checker also emphasizes the importance of trusting parental instincts. It acknowledges that parents know their children best and encourages them to seek medical care if they are concerned, even if the symptoms do not align precisely with the outlined guidelines. This personalized approach recognizes that each child is unique and may require individualized attention.

In Summary

Trusted resources and life giving information provide clear guidance as we raise our children. Seeking knowledge that resonates and holds true across credible sources is key to making sound decisions for your child. Establishing care with a consistent pediatric healthcare provider cannot be overemphasized. The pediatric medical team will learn about your child and become a trusted source of guidance. The providers are highly trained and well equipped to care for you and your child. The monitoring and advice given at the well child visits provides invaluable information and preventative measures to ensure optimal health. In addition, when your child is sick, the pediatric care team can guide you in next steps. The resources offered in this chapter are meant to supplement the information received from your primary care provider.

Our spiritual health forms the foundation of our lives, weaving through every aspect of our daily experience. As such, the Bible offers numerous passages and stories that provide hope, guidance, comfort, and praise! We are reminded of God's faithfulness, love, and His willingness to provide help to those who seek Him. Prayer allows us to express our deepest thoughts, concerns, and needs to God. It is a means to find solace, seek wisdom, strengthen our relationship with God, and worship Him. Through prayer and regular engagement with the Bible, we can find strength, hope, and wisdom in navigating life's challenges. May we draw inspiration from the words of the Bible and find comfort and confidence in the knowledge that God is our ever-present source of hope, joy, and love. Trust your God given and Holy Spirit driven intuition and seek answers to questions that linger in your heart or mind.

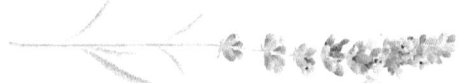

READ: *"But I trust in your mercy. Grant my heart joy in your salvation, I will sing to the Lord, for he has dealt bountifully with me!"* (Psalm 13:7)

MEDITATE: Reflect on a time when God provided you with strength or answered a prayer.

PRAY: Dear heavenly Father, open my heart to your authentic love, grace me with the strength to embrace your will, envelop my entire being with your light and joy, and fill my mind with clarity of your truth and infinite goodness. I ask all of these so that I may love you, praise you, and serve you always as your beloved daughter. Amen.

LISTEN: "House of the Lord" by Phil Wickham

RESOLVE

1. Read Psalm 100 and let thanksgiving overwhelm your heart and mind.
2. Read something from a children's Bible to your baby to remind yourself of God's Word and truth.

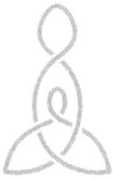

CHAPTER 9

Maximizing Sleep

"Jesus has chosen to show me the only way which leads to the Divine Furnace of love; it is the way of childlike self-surrender, the way of a child who sleeps, afraid of nothing, in its father's arms."

—St. Thérèse of Lisieux, *The Story of a Soul*

When my sons were infants, we had a small, stuffed sheep that contained a battery-operated white noise machine. The sheep went everywhere we did, and I lost count of the number of times we had to change the batteries! The soothing sounds provided a much needed element of calm. If we were visiting friends or family, the familiar background noise provided by the sheep helped ensure sweet sleep was a possibility for everyone.

I have often wondered why a sheep became the chosen animal to be associated with sleeping. Most of us are familiar with the advice to count sheep as a way to fall asleep. Perhaps the truth that Jesus is our Good Shepherd found its way into modern culture. Throughout the Bible, Our Lord promises to care for us. He does this by shepherding us back to His loving arms where we can find truth, love, and rest. I love how He does this by promising Himself to us.

"I myself will pasture my sheep; I myself will give them rest."

—Ezekiel 34:15

Rest in God

Our lives as mothers are full of beauty. However, along with the joys come endless responsibilities and countless challenges. In the midst of the busyness, God wants us to find rest. Even a great saint like Thérèse of Lisieux understood that God could come to her in sleep as a form of prayer. She wrote:

> The fact that I often fall asleep during meditation, or while making my thanksgiving, should appall me. Well, I am not appalled; I bear in mind that little children are just as pleasing to their parents asleep as awake; that doctors put their patients to sleep while they perform operations; and that after all, *"the Lord knoweth our frame. He remembereth that we are but dust"* (Psalm 102:14).[48]

Jesus offers us solace, rejuvenation, and strength in His presence. We are not alone in our journey. We are promised support and love. He calls us to place our burdens and worries in His loving arms and receive comfort and peace. Resting in Jesus enables us to tap into His limitless grace and wisdom, seeking His guidance and relying on His strength to navigate the joys and struggles of motherhood. We can find renewed purpose and perspective, keeping our focus on eternal values and the significance of our roles in shaping the lives of our children.

We are reminded of our identity as beloved daughters of God, cherished and valued for who we are, not for what we do.

---

48   Thérèse of Lisieux, *Story of a Soul: The Autobiography of St. Thérèse of Lisieux*, translated by Michael Day, translator (Charlotte, NC: Saint Benedict Press, 2010), 97.

As we journey through life, we can be comforted that God is always with us. For example, when Moses was in need of assurance and guidance, God promised to be with him and grant him rest: "The Lord answered: I myself will go along, to give you rest" (Exodus 33:14). This verse reminds us that intentionally placing ourselves in the presence of God brings an opportunity for rest. We can do this wherever we are, however we look, and in whatever emotional or mental state we may be in. We simply call out for God to be with us. His comforting and strengthening presence brings solace to our weary souls, offering a deep and lasting rest that surpasses any worldly understanding.

"Come to me, all you who labor and are burdened, and I will give you rest. Take my yoke upon you and learn from me, for I am meek and humble of heart; and you will find rest for yourselves. For my yoke is easy, and my burden light."

—Matthew 11:28–30

Jesus invites all who are weary and burdened to come to Him. As we learn from Him, we will discover rest for our souls. Jesus offers a gentle and compassionate approach, lightening our burdens and providing a peaceful refuge. By seeking His presence, learning from Him, and trusting in His care, we can experience a profound sense of peace and rest in the midst of the challenges of motherhood and life in general. This is a real, tangible peace that comes only from God!

And when we stray, He comes after us! He is determined for us to be with Him.

"What is your opinion? If a man has a hundred sheep and one of them goes astray, will he not leave the ninety-nine in the hills and go in search of the stray?

And if he finds it, amen, I say to you, he rejoices more
over it than over the ninety-nine that did not stray.
In just the same way, it is not the will of your heavenly
Father that one of these little ones be lost."

—Matthew 18:12–14

Normal Sleeping Patterns

Everyone in the family needs restorative rest and sleep. For infants, adequate sleep is vital for their optimal overall development. Rapid brain development occurs during the first three years of life, and sleep plays a crucial role. Sleep is foundational for the growth of neurological functions such as memory, learning, and emotional regulation. Understanding normal sleep patterns and what to expect can help navigate this important aspect of health. Sleep patterns and individual variations are common, but there are some general guidelines. Also note that babies may have growth spurts, sleep regressions, or periods of increased fussiness that can temporarily disrupt their sleep patterns. Always use safe sleep guidelines by placing infants on their backs to sleep, using a firm mattress, and avoiding loose bedding or toys in the crib.

The First Twelve Weeks

Bonding, attachment, and responsiveness are essential during a baby's first twelve weeks of life. It's true when people say you cannot "spoil" a baby by holding them and answering their cries at this age. Your newborn is learning that they can trust you to respond to their cries. Placing the crib or bassinet in your room will help you respond to your infant in a timely way. Also, it helps optimize you getting back into your bed for sleep as well!

NEWBORNS (ZERO TO FOUR WEEKS):

Irregular sleep patterns are to be expected at this age, with total sleeping time of approximately fourteen to seventeen hours per day. This sleep often occurs in short bursts. Babies typically wake every two to three hours to feed, and their sleep/awake cycles are shorter, ranging from thirty minutes to three hours. Newborns are born with a startle reflex (also called the Moro reflex) that gradually goes away typically between four to six months of age. Though normal, this reflex can sometimes disrupt infants' sleep. To prevent your baby from startling themselves awake, you may consider swaddling your baby. Swaddling can be helpful as this mimics being in your womb and may help your baby feel secure and comforted. If you choose to swaddle, keep in mind that swaddling should be done with a thin blanket and your baby should be able to freely move their hips when swaddled. Never use weighted blankets or swaddles with your infant and ensure they are not overheated when swaddled.[49]

ONE TO TWO MONTHS:

As babies grow, they may start developing longer periods of sleep at night, with some stretches lasting four to six hours. Daytime naps may range from thirty minutes to two or three hours. If you are breastfeeding, don't be concerned if your infant does not sleep these longer stretches yet!

TWO TO THREE MONTHS:

By this stage, some infants may sleep for longer stretches at night, with some managing five to six hours without waking. Total sleep is around twelve to sixteen hours per day, including two to five naps of varying lengths.

---

49   Rachel Y. Moon, MD, FAAP, and Danette Glassy, MD, FAAP, "Swaddling: Is It Safe?",
      HealthyChildren.org, accessed May 6, 2025, https://www.healthychildren.org/English/ages-stages/
      baby/diapers-clothing/Pages/Swaddling-Is-it-Safe.aspx.

This is also the expected age of PURPLE crying (as discussed in chapter 3). Once you have responded to your infant's needs of feeding, soothing, and diapering, remember that it's okay to place them in a safe sleeping location and walk away to give yourself an opportunity to calm and recenter.

There are studies that indicate that pacifier use may protect infants from SIDS (sudden infant death syndrome). Because of this protective effect, the American Academy of Pediatrics recommends offering babies pacifiers at nap and bedtime. If your baby does not take a pacifier or spits out the pacifier after they fall asleep, you don't need to replace it. You may wait until breastfeeding is established before offering a pacifier. And don't attach the pacifier to your infant's clothing or put it around their neck.

Between two to four months, it's time to start weaning your baby from a swaddle. By the time babies start to roll over, swaddling should be completely discontinued. While infants may continue to wear a sleep sack for warmth if needed, they should have their arms free at this time.[50]

MONTHS THREE TO SIX

During the three to six months stage, infants begin to establish more predictable sleep patterns. Infants at this age typically require around fourteen to sixteen hours of sleep per day, including naps and nighttime sleep. During this stage, most babies will begin to sleep for longer stretches during the night, ranging from nine to ten hours. However, it can be normal for them to wake up one or two times, especially for feedings. Infants three to six months old will often take two to four naps during the day, adding up to a total of four to five hours of sleep.[51] During this time, babies may start developing self-

---

50   Moon and Glassy, "Swaddling: Is It Safe?"

51   "Infant Sleep," Children's Hospital of Philadelphia, accessed May 7, 2025, https://www.chop.edu/primary-care/infant-sleep.

soothing skills. They may be able to fall asleep on their own without needing to be rocked or fed to sleep. Encouraging self-soothing can help promote independent sleep. Responding to your infant for feeding and soothing during this age is dependent on your child's unique needs and your own circumstances. Please consult your pediatric healthcare provider for individualized sleep advice.

MONTHS SIX TO TWELVE

During six to twelve months, babies typically continue to refine their sleep patterns, gradually moving toward a more structured sleep schedule. However, each child is unique, and sleep patterns can vary.

Most babies within this age range still require around twelve to fifteen hours of sleep per day, which includes nighttime sleep and daytime naps. Nighttime sleep may consist of approximately ten to twelve hours, with the ability to sleep for longer stretches without needing to feed.

At this stage, babies often begin to establish more regular sleep routines, with three naps gradually transitioning into one to two naps. These naps can range from one to two hours each, although the duration may vary from child to child.

It's common for infants in this age group to experience some night wakings. Helping them develop self-soothing skills will allow them to return to sleep independently.

It's also common for infants to experience sleep regressions, where their sleep patterns temporarily become disrupted. These regressions can be triggered by developmental milestones, growth spurts, or changes in routine. Patience and consistency during these periods are key.

While these sleep patterns serve as a general guide, individual variations are common. Each child develops at their own pace, and their sleep needs may differ. If you have concerns about your child's sleep patterns or if they consistently have trouble falling asleep or staying asleep, we recommend consulting with a pediatric healthcare provider for personalized guidance and support.

Sleep for Baby: Practical Tips

- **Follow a consistent routine:** Establish a predictable sleep routine by creating a consistent sequence of activities before bedtime. Ideas to consider include a warm bath, soothing massage, singing lullabies, reading a book, or saying prayers. Consistency helps signal to your baby that it's time to wind down and prepares them for sleep.

- **Create a conducive sleep environment:** Ensure your baby's sleep space is safe, comfortable, and conducive to sleep. Keep the room dark and at a comfortable temperature; your level of dress and comfort is a good guide. Use a firm crib mattress with a fitted sheet. Don't use bumper pads, loose bedding, or stuffed animals, as these are associated with risks of suffocation. A white noise machine is helpful to provide a sound for your baby to focus on as other household noises are happening. We intentionally did not require absolute silence in our home because we wanted the boys to learn to sleep more readily in a variety of environments.

- **Encourage self-soothing:** As babies grow, they can gradually develop self-soothing skills. Give your baby the opportunity to fall asleep independently by putting them down when they're drowsy but awake. This can help them learn to self-settle and go back to sleep if they wake during the night. Using a pacifier or allowing thumb/finger sucking can be a helpful soothing technique. Do not offer a bottle in the bed. Not only is there a risk for choking, but it also contributes to ear infections, changes in mouth formation, and oral cavities later in life.

- HELPFUL TIP: Once our sons were moved to their own room, I used to sit on the floor next to their crib to say their nighttime prayers. I would then remind them of all of the people who loved them. Once they were calm, I would slowly leave their rooms, telling them they were loved and guarded by God as I walked out.

- **Establish daytime and nighttime differences:** Create a distinction between daytime and nighttime sleep by exposing your baby to natural light and engaging in stimulating activities during the day. During nighttime feedings or diaper changes, slightly dim the room. Putting a dimmer switch in the bedroom was one of the best investments we made.

- **Be mindful of sleep cues:** Watch for signs of sleepiness such as yawning, rubbing their eyes, or becoming fussy. Putting your baby down for sleep when they show these cues helps prevent overtiredness and makes it easier for them to fall asleep.

- **Monitor awake times:** Pay attention to your baby's awake times (often referred to as their "wake window") and make sure they are getting enough sleep overall. As they grow, their awake times will lengthen, and their nap schedule may evolve. Observe their sleep patterns and adjust accordingly to ensure they are well-rested. Understanding and following age-appropriate wake windows can help prevent overtiredness and make naps and nighttime sleep more restful and predictable.

- **Consider using infant equipment:** Our youngest loved his swing! He enjoyed a birthday celebration from his swing. However, when he fell asleep, we moved him to his crib as sleeping in a swing is a risk for suffocation. Always ensure your baby is strapped into any seat, swing, or device you put them in. Check for any recalls on infant equipment as suffocation has been associated with some equipment. Ensure an adult is present, awake, and attentive and moves the baby to a crib if the baby falls asleep. Baby carriers are another popular option. Be sure to follow the instructions and weight requirements and use the carrier properly. Also, monitor how your baby responds to being in a carrier. While this was an excellent option for my two sons, this is a personal decision, and you will find what works best for you.

Remember, every baby is unique, and it will take time to establish consistent sleep and rest patterns. Be patient, flexible, and open to adjusting your approach as needed. What works for one baby may not work for the next baby, and what works for one family may not work for another. If you have concerns about your baby's sleep or rest, consult with a pediatric healthcare provider for personalized guidance and support.

Sleep for Mom: Practical Tips

Getting enough rest and sleep will be challenging, but it's crucial for your well-being. Creating an intentional plan for sleep and then adjusting as you and your baby's needs change will help maximize this crucial component of health. Here are practical tips to help promote better sleep and rest:

- **Prioritize sleep:** Recognize the importance of your own sleep and make it a priority. When your baby sleeps, try to nap or rest as well, even if it's for short intervals. The most challenging part is learning what tasks are not absolutely necessary and letting them go. With my first baby, I learned this the hard way! I kept pushing myself, and my episiotomy was not healing. It took a doctor ordering me to take a sitz bath four times a day before I allowed myself to rest. Once I let go of nonessential tasks, got better at asking for help, and rested my body, I was better able to respond to my infant. I learned to put a diaper-changing station and bassinet in the living room, and when my son started to show signs of being ready for a nap, I quickly ensured he had a dry diaper, swaddled him, and laid him in the bassinet. Then I would lie down on the couch and try to get whatever rest I could.

- **Share responsibilities:** Enlist the help of your partner, family members, or trusted friends to share baby care duties. This allows you to have designated periods for uninterrupted sleep or rest. Communicate your needs and seek support when needed.

- **Establish a sleep-friendly environment and bedtime routine:** Ensure your sleep environment is comfortable, safe, and conducive to sleep. I was amazed at how quickly our bedroom became cluttered with baby gear, clothes (both clean and dirty!), and miscellaneous gifts. Keeping the bedroom organized and establishing a new routine for laundry was a priority as this helped create a calm environment for my husband, myself, and our baby. We also needed to establish a new bedtime routine even though we knew we would be awake again in two hours! This helped our bodies know sleep was the next activity. Invest in blackout curtains, eye covers, and white noise machines to create a soothing ambiance.

- **Practice prayer:** Take time for self-care activities that promote relaxation and reduce stress. Meditative prayer or repetitive prayers such as the Rosary or Divine Mercy Chaplet help to focus your mind and reconnect with God. Repeat a selected Bible verse to remind yourself of God's goodness. Consider guided meditation using an app or podcast of your choice. Hallow is a favorite of mine and offers a wide variety of options. Remember, a well-rested and rejuvenated mother is better equipped to care for her baby.

- **Rest counts:** Sometimes I would lie down to take a nap,
  but sleep would not come. Over time, I learned not to trade
  that moment for chores but instead read or take extra time
  cuddling and rocking my baby. These quiet moments of
  timelessness rested my mind and body and soothed my soul.

Be patient with yourself and your baby as you navigate the journey of
sleep and rest. If you have concerns about your baby's sleep or you're
experiencing persistent sleep deprivation or anxiety, don't hesitate
to reach out to your healthcare provider for guidance and support.

The Opinions of Others

You can expect to hear quite a bit from others about their opinions
relating to sleep and rest for you and your new baby. When it comes
to receiving and listening to advice from others during the first
twelve months, approach this with an open mind and discernment.
Here are a few points to consider:

- **Seek advice from trusted sources:** Recognize that not all
  advice will be applicable or beneficial to your situation.
  Consider the context, evaluate the advice critically, and choose
  what aligns with your parenting style and values. Consult
  reliable healthcare professionals, experienced parents, or
  reputable sources for information and guidance. Consider the
  credibility and expertise of the person offering advice.

- **Remember that every baby is unique:** What works for one
  baby may not work for another. Each child has their own
  temperament, preferences, and needs. Keep in mind that
  advice should be tailored to your specific situation and adapted
  accordingly.

- **Trust your discernment:** As a mother, you possess a natural
  intuition when it comes to your baby. Trust your prayerful

intuition in making decisions about your baby's sleep and rest routines. Communicate early and often with your spouse about sleeping routines. Partnering on this essential element of health can help optimize sleep for everyone.

- **Prioritize your baby's safety and well-being:** Follow evidence-based guidelines and recommendations, such as safe sleep practices, to ensure a secure sleep environment. Ultimately, as a mother, you are the expert on your own child. Listen to advice with an open mind, filter it through your own knowledge and intuition, and make decisions that best support your baby's health and well-being. If you are experiencing challenges with your baby's sleep or rest, consult with a healthcare professional or pediatrician. They can provide personalized guidance and support tailored to your baby's unique needs.

Resources

In addition to the American Academy of Pediatrics, the following resources provide reputable and reliable information to support parents in understanding and addressing their baby's sleep and rest needs. It's wise to consider multiple sources and consult with healthcare professionals for personalized advice based on your baby's unique circumstances.

- The National Sleep Foundation (NSF) offers guidance and resources for promoting healthy sleep habits for all ages, including infants. Their website (**www.sleepfoundation.org**) provides articles, tips, and educational materials to support parents in understanding and establishing healthy sleep routines for their babies.

- Baby Sleep Science (**www.babysleepscience.com**) is a trusted resource created by sleep experts that provides evidence-based information and strategies for parents seeking to understand and address their baby's sleep patterns. They offer helpful articles, sleep training methods, and personalized sleep consulting services.

- Precious Little Sleep (**www.preciouslittlesleep.com**) is a popular website and book by Alexis Dubief, providing practical advice and evidence-based strategies for improving infant and toddler sleep. Both offer a wealth of information, including sleep schedules, sleep training techniques, and troubleshooting tips.

In Summary

In the midst of our selfless acts of love and sacrifice, we need moments of rest in Jesus to be replenished, refreshed, and filled with the divine peace that surpasses understanding. It is in this rest that we can experience the strength necessary to embrace our calling as mothers with grace, resilience, and joy. God encourages us to call on Him throughout our day, in all that we do.

The words of Psalm 127:2 remind us that "it is vain for you to rise early and put off your rest at night, to eat bread earned by hard toil— all this God gives to his beloved in sleep."

As you work to establish healthy sleep patterns for your baby, remember that God provides the same care and guidance for you. The practical tips for infant sleep outlined in this chapter work best when balanced with your own rest and prayer time. Take a moment each day to pause, breathe, and ask God for the strength and wisdom you need. Both you and your baby will benefit from this intentional combination of practical and spiritual care.

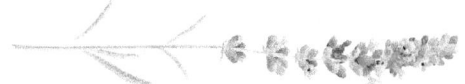

READ: *"Where you saw how the Lord, your God, carried you, as one carries his own child, all along your journey until you arrived at this place."* (Deuteronomy 1:31)

MEDITATE: Imagine God carrying you just like you carry your baby.

PRAY: "O Jesus, I surrender myself to You; take care of everything!" —Father Dolindo Ruotolo, *The Surrender Novena*

CONTEMPLATE: How is God calling you to carve out time in your day for rest?

LISTEN: "Rest in You" by All Sons and Daughters

RESOLVE: Decide on one action you can take to create an opportunity for rest.

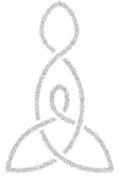

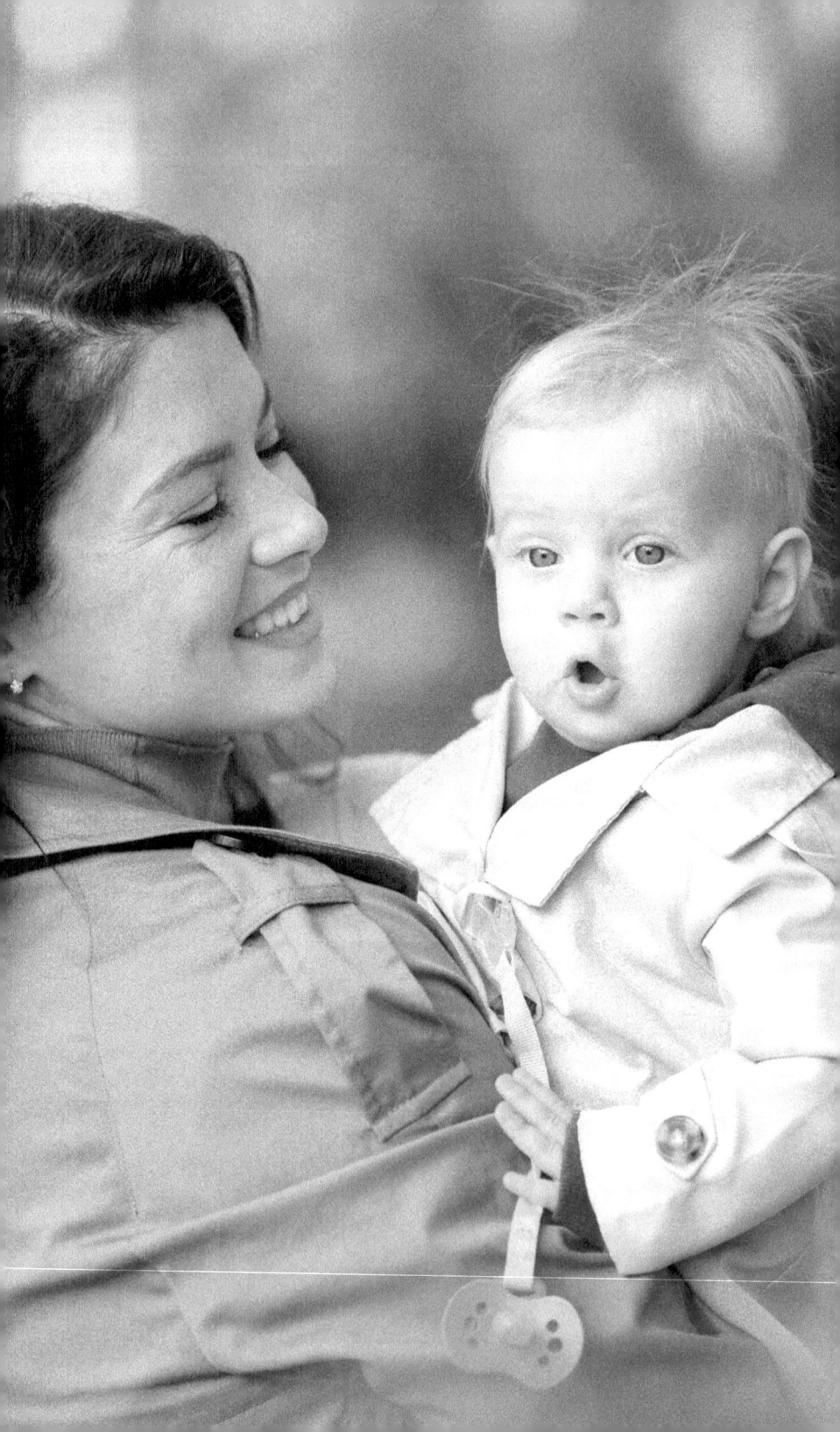

CHAPTER 10

Adapting to Life
with Baby

The morning after our youngest was born, my husband went to the hospital cafeteria to get some breakfast tacos and coffee while I enjoyed some quiet moments alone with our baby boy. As I snuggled and gazed at him, my heart was full of joy and awe. I knew our lives had changed in a beautiful and profound way. However, it wasn't until that first drive home that it really sunk in! Once we arrived at our house and I was settling into the nursery chair to breastfeed, I prayed that God would stay near and guide our changing lives.

> *"I came so that they might have life and have it more abundantly."*
>
> —John 10:10

St. John encapsulates in this beautiful verse the essence of Christ's mission: to offer a life enriched with meaning, purpose, and joy. His will is for us to live abundantly, but not as the world suggests. Instead, He wants us to grow in His love and desires our spiritual lives be firmly planted in His nurturing garden. The joyful transition of welcoming a newborn into your home and life is accompanied with increased daily demands. Jesus wants us to stay close to Him and be transformed according to His will.

Jesus Is the Vine, and We Are the Branches

Jesus often used metaphors and parables to convey profound spiritual truths. One such metaphor is the depiction of Himself as the vine and His followers as the branches. This analogy highlights the intimate and life-giving relationship between Jesus and His disciples, and it also offers a unique insight into the role of mothers in the spiritual journey.

In the Gospel of John, Jesus declared, "I am the true vine, and my Father is the vine grower" (John 15:1). By referring to Himself as the "true vine," Jesus implied that He is the authentic source of life and nourishment for His followers. Just as a vine sustains and nurtures its branches, Jesus provides spiritual sustenance, guidance, and support to those who abide in Him.

When Jesus speaks of us as the branches, He emphasizes our role as bearers and nurturers of life. Just as branches receive their life and sustenance from the vine, moms draw their strength and wisdom from their connection to Jesus. We are entrusted with the precious responsibility of nurturing and shaping the lives of our children, instilling in them the values of love, compassion, and faith.

"Remain in me, as I remain in you. Just as a branch cannot bear fruit on its own unless it remains on the vine, so neither can you unless you remain in me. I am the vine, you are the branches. Whoever remains in me and I in him will bear much fruit, because without me you can do nothing."

—John 15:4–5

These verses emphasize the importance of staying connected to Jesus, just as branches cannot grow if they are not attached to the vine. By abiding in Jesus, we find the strength and grace we need to fulfill our vital role. It is through our union with Christ that we can bear spiritual fruit in our lives and positively influence our children and families.

We are recipients of and conduits for God's love and grace. In John 15:9–10, Jesus said, "As the Father loves me, so I also love you. Remain in my love. If you keep my commandments, you will remain in my love, just as I have kept my Father's commandments and remain in his love." Here, Jesus underscored the importance of love and obedience in the life of His followers. Similarly, mothers are called to embody God's love in their relationships with their children and others. By remaining in Christ's love, they can extend that love to their families, fostering an environment of love, harmony, and spiritual growth.

Furthermore, Jesus assured His disciples that their connection to Him as the vine grants them access to the power of prayer. In John 15:7, He said, "If you remain in me and my words remain in you, ask for whatever you want and it will be done for you." This promise holds true for us as well. Through our abiding relationship with Jesus, we can approach God with confidence, seeking guidance, wisdom, and strength to fulfill our maternal duties. We can rely on God's faithfulness to provide for our needs and to work through us for the well-being of our children.

The metaphor of Jesus as the vine and mothers as the branches beautifully illustrates how we depend on Christ while nurturing our children's lives. Through our connection to Jesus, we receive the spiritual nourishment, strength, and guidance we need to fulfill our roles as mothers effectively. By abiding in Christ's love and obeying His commands, we can bear spiritual fruit in our lives and pass on the values of love, compassion, and faith to the next generation.

Day-to-Day Realities

Bringing a newborn home is an awe-inspiring and transformative experience for any new mother. However, amid the joy and love, it also presents a multitude of challenges and adjustments as she navigates the uncharted waters of motherhood. The initial days and weeks after returning home with a baby are filled with a mix of emotions, physical demands, and lifestyle changes that can be overwhelming and exhausting.

First, juggling household responsibilities with the demands of a newborn is challenging. The laundry piles up, dishes accumulate, and tidying the house might seem like an impossible task. Many new mothers struggle with the desire to maintain a clean and organized home while also devoting time to their baby's care.

Feeding challenges can also arise shortly after bringing your new baby home. Whether a mother chooses to breastfeed or use formula, feeding a newborn can be demanding. Breastfeeding requires patience, practice, and often comes with its own set of difficulties such as latching issues, sore nipples, and concerns about milk supply. On the other hand, formula feeding involves the preparation of bottles, cleaning of bottles, and ensuring the baby is getting the right amount of nutrition. Additionally, some babies may experience colic or reflux, adding to the complexity of feeding routines.

New mothers also quickly learn that time is now a precious commodity. Caring for a newborn can consume a significant portion of the day, leaving little time for other tasks. Simple activities such as eating, showering, or getting dressed need to be carefully planned around the baby's schedule. Time management becomes a vital skill for new mothers to ensure they meet their own needs while tending to their baby's demands.

Though new moms face these adjustments and challenges, we can find inspiration from Saint Thérèse of Lisieux. Also known as the "Little Flower of Jesus," Saint Thérèse is renowned for her unique approach to spirituality, which she termed "the little way." Born in 1873, Thérèse grew up in a devout Catholic family in France. Despite facing personal challenges, including the loss of her mother at a young age and her own fragile health, she developed a deep love for God and a desire to serve Him. At the age of fifteen, she entered the Carmelite convent in Lisieux. In the convent, Thérèse practiced this "little way" by embracing tasks that were often overlooked or undervalued, such as helping her fellow sisters or offering up her daily struggles and inconveniences as acts of love to God. She believed that these small acts, done with love, were highly valued in the eyes of God. Her "little way" demonstrates that true freedom in Christ is found not in grandiose actions but in loving as He loved, in the ordinary and everyday routines.

KATHRYN

My three years of pediatric residency and two as a private practice pediatrician did not prepare me for those initial nights home with our first daughter! My husband and I both distinctly remember the first few nights. My milk was not in yet and, as is common with newborns, my daughter had her days and nights mixed up. After attempting to breastfeed her, she was still wide awake and fussy. I remember my husband and I staring at each other, wondering what to do! We both ended up staying up almost all night trying to get her to sleep. We quickly learned that was not sustainable! We then developed a plan to divide the night into shifts. After I was done breastfeeding, if it was not my shift, I would go back to sleep, and my husband would take the baby. If it was my shift, my husband would sleep until the next feed. This was much more practical and allowed each of us to at least get a couple of hours of sleep! When our second and third babies were born, we automatically fell into this routine and laughed about how little we knew with our first!

Plan to Succeed

There isn't one right way to adjust to having a new baby! But there are a few recommendations for helping you make a plan to succeed.

Establishing a structured routine for your baby's daily activities, such as feeding, sleeping, and playtime, can help you adapt. This helps establish a sense of predictability and makes it easier for everyone involved to contribute. Early on, babies may not follow a precise routine; that's normal and almost expected. Even if your baby does not follow a strict schedule, you can still establish a routine for yourself.

While routines are essential, flexibility is equally important. Adapt the schedule to your baby's changing needs and growth stages. Stay patient—it might take time for routines to settle in. A well-established routine brings comfort and balance to both mother and child, leading to a more harmonious and enjoyable motherhood experience.

Planning to succeed also means taking time to care for yourself too. Take breaks, rest when you can, and engage in activities that rejuvenate you. Self-care ensures you have the energy and mental well-being to be the best mother you can be.

Part of any plan to succeed also includes making sure you have adequate support. The challenges of new motherhood can be emotionally and physically draining, making it essential for mothers to seek support from their partners, family, or friends. Building a support network provides new mothers with reassurance, practical help, and opportunities to share their experiences and concerns with others who understand. Below we highlight some things to consider when building your support network.

Amid the challenges, the day-to-day realities of motherhood also include moments of pure joy and bonding with your baby. The first smile, coo, or milestone achieved brings immense happiness and a sense of fulfillment. These precious moments serve as a reminder of the incredible gift of motherhood and make the trials worthwhile.

TEAMWORK MAKES THE DREAM WORK

As mentioned above, having a good support network can dramatically improve daily life. Embracing the motto "teamwork makes the dream work" can help you navigate the joys and challenges of motherhood more smoothly. Here is some advice to keep in mind:

- **Communicate openly:** Share your thoughts, concerns, and needs with your spouse, family, and friends. Effective communication builds a strong support system and allows others to understand how they can help. Be open about your needs and expectations, ensuring everyone understands their role. Clarity is kind! Communicate the specific tasks or areas where you require assistance.

- **Set boundaries:** Respectfully express when you need personal space or time with your baby. Setting boundaries prevents misunderstandings, promotes a healthy support system, and allows you to maintain your autonomy as a mother.

- **Delegate responsibilities:** Don't hesitate to ask for help when you need it. Delegate tasks like diaper changes, feeding, or household chores to your spouse, family members, or trusted friends. Sharing the load promotes a sense of togetherness.

- **Support each other emotionally:** Parenthood can be overwhelming, so be there for your partner and allow them to be there for you. Offer a listening ear, validate each other's experiences, and provide emotional support during challenging moments.

Don't hesitate to seek assistance from others when needed. Asking for help doesn't make you weak; it showcases strength and wisdom in recognizing your limitations. Reach out to your partner, family, or friends for support in parenting, household chores, or emotional well-being. Accepting help enables you to recharge and prevents burnout. Remember, you are not alone in this journey. Lean on your support system, share the joys and challenges, and allow others to be there for you. Seeking assistance doesn't diminish your role as a mother; it enhances your ability to provide the best care and love to your child. Embrace the power of community, and together, you can thrive in motherhood.

COMMUNITY RESOURCES

In addition to your close family and friends, be sure to explore the wealth of community resources available to assist you with your children. Many local organizations offer parenting classes, support groups, and workshops that provide valuable insights and guidance. Reach out to public libraries for story-time sessions or to borrow educational materials. Check with community centers or churches for child care services or playgroups where your child can socialize and learn. Look into government programs for financial aid, healthcare, and early childhood education. Online forums and social media groups can also connect you with other parents, fostering a supportive virtual community. Utilize these resources to ease the challenges of motherhood, gain knowledge, and build lasting connections within your community. Here is some advice on tapping into these valuable resources:

- **Religious organizations:** Churches often provide valuable assistance for mothers and their children. They may offer child care during services or events, giving moms a chance to participate while ensuring their child's safety and care. Some churches organize support groups or parenting classes, creating a space for moms to connect, share experiences, and receive guidance. Additionally, churches often organize community outreach programs that provide resources such as food, clothing, and educational support for children in need.

- **Parenting support groups:** Join local parenting support groups or online communities where you can connect with other mothers. These groups offer a safe space to share experiences, seek advice, and build lasting friendships.

- **Public libraries:** Public libraries often host story times, playgroups, and educational events for children. Take advantage of these resources to engage your child in learning and socializing with other kids.

- **Community centers:** Check out community centers that offer child-friendly activities and workshops. As your baby grows, they might have programs for arts and crafts, music, sports, and more.

- **Healthcare services:** Utilize healthcare services like pediatric clinics and maternal support programs. These services provide guidance on child development, nutrition, and health-related concerns.

- **Parenting workshops:** Attend parenting workshops or seminars to enhance your parenting skills and gain valuable insights from experts.

- **Child-care services:** If you need occasional child care, explore local daycare centers or certified babysitters who can look after your child when you have appointments or commitments.

- **Hotlines and helplines:** Familiarize yourself with hotlines and helplines that provide parenting advice or emotional support during challenging times.

- **Government assistance programs:** If finances are tight, look into government assistance programs that offer financial aid, child care vouchers, or other resources.

Seeking help from community resources doesn't imply inadequacy. It's a proactive step toward creating a strong support network, enriching your child's life, and enhancing your own well-being as a mother. Embrace these resources, and let them be a valuable asset in your parenting journey.

Returning to Work

Returning to work after having a baby presents new moms with a host of challenges. Balancing the demands of their career and the needs of their newborn can lead to feelings of guilt and stress. Separation anxiety, especially during the initial days, adds emotional strain. Juggling breastfeeding or pumping at work can be physically demanding and time-consuming. Sleep deprivation from caring for the baby at night can impact job performance. Navigating workplace policies and support for working mothers can be confusing and frustrating. Overall, the transition back to work can be overwhelming as new moms strive to find a harmonious work-life balance.

- **Plan and practice your routine:** Before your first day back at work, try practicing your new routine a few times. This includes waking up early, getting ready, preparing for your baby's needs, and figuring out your commute. This practice can help alleviate some stress and give you a clearer idea of how much time you will need each morning.

- **Communicate with your employer:** Have an open and honest conversation with your employer about your needs and any adjustments to your schedule that might be necessary. This might include discussing flexible hours, remote work options, or a phased return to work. Employers are increasingly understanding of the needs of new parents, and having this conversation early can help set expectations on both sides.

- **Set realistic goals and expectations:** Accept that it might take some time to get back into the swing of things at work. Be patient with yourself and set realistic expectations about what you can achieve as you balance work and motherhood. Remember that it's okay not to be perfect and takes time to find the right balance.

- **Establish a support system:** Having a strong support system is crucial. This could include your partner, family, friends, or a nanny. They can assist with child care, household chores, or simply offer emotional support. Additionally, connecting with other working moms, either in your workplace or in social groups, can provide valuable advice and understanding.

- **Prioritize self-care:** Don't forget to take care of yourself. It's easy to get caught up in the demands of being a new mom and an employee, but your well-being is essential. This can mean setting aside time for exercise, ensuring you get enough sleep, or even just finding a few minutes a day to relax and recharge.

- **Plan for breastfeeding or pumping:** If you're planning to continue breastfeeding, ask your employer about having a private space where you can pump. Invest in a good quality breast pump and learn how to store breast milk properly. It's also helpful to start pumping and storing milk a few weeks before returning to work to build up a supply. Additionally, wearing comfortable, breastfeeding-friendly clothes to work can make the process easier. Your right to pump at work is protected by federal law, so don't hesitate to advocate for your needs.

Remember, every new mom's experience is unique, so what works for one person may not work for another. It is important to find what best suits you and your family's needs.

Staying Home

When I decided to transition from my job to staying at home, I realized I had unconsciously assigned my identity to my profession. Once at home, I poured into my family physically and emotionally, but my intellectual abilities were no longer being challenged in the same way as when I was practicing nursing. This realization contributed to some depression at first, but then it made me realize I had some work to do spiritually. Being at home was a huge gift that taught me to realign how I defined my self-worth. The opportunity also taught my children to know that *who* they are is what is important, not *what* they do.

Transitioning from a career to being a stay-at-home mom is a profound shift, but remember that your identity is not defined by your job or your role at home. Your identity is founded in the truth that you are a daughter of the One True King! Here are five tips to help you navigate this transition with confidence and faith:

1. **Root your identity in Christ:** Your worth is not based on your productivity or achievements but on who you are in God's eyes. Spend time in prayer and Scripture to remind yourself that you are loved, chosen, and called for a purpose, whether in the workplace or at home.

2. **Build a faith-filled community:** Surround yourself with other faith-driven women who can encourage and uplift you. Join a Bible study, mom's group, or church community to stay connected and grow spiritually during this season.

3. **Establish a grace-filled routine:** While structure is helpful, allow yourself grace when things don't go as planned. Incorporate prayer and quiet time into your daily routine to keep your heart centered on Christ.

4. **Communicate and trust God's provision:** Keep an open dialogue with your spouse about responsibilities and finances, trusting that God will provide for your family's needs. Lean on Him for wisdom and strength in managing your home.

5. **Prioritize self-care through faith:** Taking care of yourself spiritually, emotionally, and physically allows you to pour into your family. Make time for worship, personal growth, and rest, knowing that God equips you for this calling.

Embrace this season with joy, knowing that your ultimate purpose is to serve the Lord in whatever role He calls you to. Ultimately, transitioning from career to home requires adaptation, support, and self-compassion to navigate the challenges and embrace a new, fulfilling role.

Safe Child Care

Keith and I agreed that Charlie would be at home with me or a nanny for the first nine to twelve months. We wanted to get through the cold and flu season before putting him in daycare. My sister agreed to be with me while interviewing nannies, and having two sets of eyes and ears on the person made me more comfortable. One particular lady seemed to have the right references, the right experience, the right personality, and the right price. However, my sister and I just knew something was off. The background check revealed she had a questionable financial history and had been convicted of vandalism. This was a clear answer that she was not the right person to be caring for our child. We ultimately found a lovely nanny that fit perfectly with our family and baby, and we are forever grateful. Take the time and pay the cost of background checks before allowing someone to take care of your child.

Choosing the right child care for your children is a significant decision that requires careful consideration. Whether you're returning to work or just need occasional support, finding a nurturing and safe environment is essential. We have included some advice to help you make an informed choice in Appendix 3.

In Summary

The day-to-day realities after returning home with your baby are a complex tapestry of emotions, physical demands, and lifestyle adjustments. From sleep deprivation and feeding challenges to the emotional roller coaster and lack of personal time, you may feel as if you're facing numerous hurdles. However, amid these difficulties, you can also experience the joy and bonding that come with nurturing a new life.

The journey of motherhood is life-changing, filled with both challenges and rewards. Through perseverance, support, and self-care, we know you will find the strength to embrace this new chapter. This strength, drawn from family, friends, community, and faith, creates the foundation upon which abundant life can flourish. As Jesus teaches us that He came so we might have life abundantly, motherhood offers a unique window into this divine abundance.

In the small, everyday moments of caring for your baby you participate in St. Therese's "little way," offering these little acts of love as prayer. The unconditional love you develop for your child deepens your understanding of God's love for you. Embracing motherhood with faith allows this season to become not just a period of adjustment, but a holy journey where challenges and joys together create something beautiful in God's eyes.

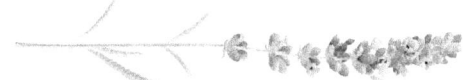

READ: *"Miss no single opportunity of making some small sacrifice, here by a smiling look, there by a kindly word; always doing the smallest right and doing it all for love."* — St. Thérèse of Lisieux

MEDITATE: In the ordinary moments of caring for your baby, reflect on how each small act—offered with love—can be offered as a sacred prayer.

PRAY: Sometimes when I am in such a state of spiritual dryness that not a single good thought occurs to me, I say very slowly the "Our Father," or the "Hail Mary," and these prayers suffice to take me out of myself. —St. Thérèse of Lisieux

LISTEN: "Lord, I Need You" by Matt Maher

RESOLVE

1. Wear a bracelet, pin, or other accessory that reminds you to pray throughout your day.
2. Intentionally offer up a chore you dislike doing as a prayer.

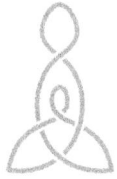

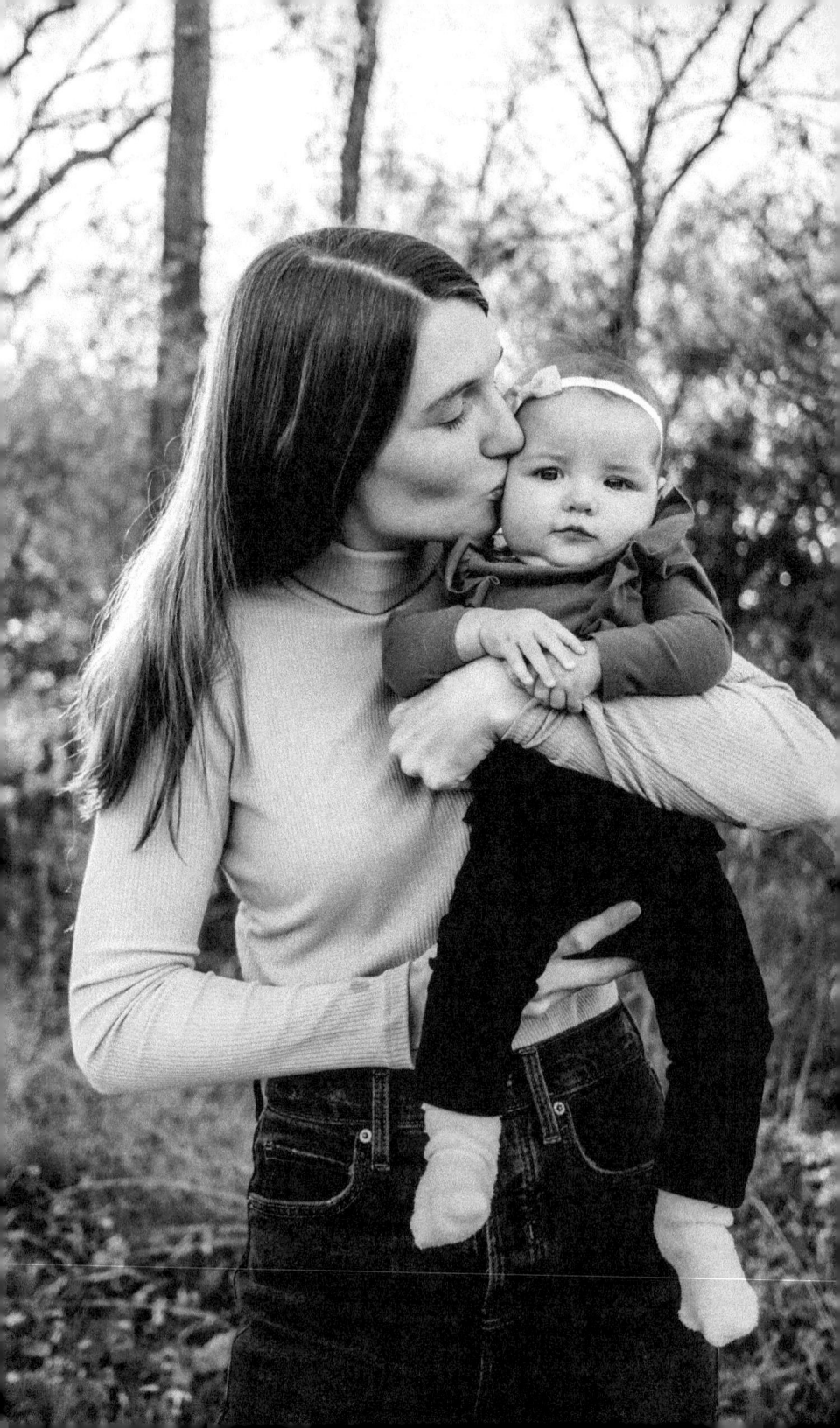

CHAPTER 11

Self-Care

As I was getting on the elevator to go home after a particularly difficult and long day taking care of patients, a fellow nurse practitioner asked me, "What does taking care of myself even mean?" My initial response was a tired "eating healthy and getting sleep." She and I both chuckled, knowing neither of us made the best snack choices when 3:00 p.m. rolled around!

I have thought of this question often in my life, and writing this chapter has been challenging. After much prayer and reflection on my own experiences and the choices I've made, along with their consequences, I hope these words resonate with you. What self-care means to you is deeply personal and may change over time. But it's important to recognize that true self-care is an ongoing journey with spiritual growth at its core.

In a recent session, my counselor said to me, "It's good that you are able to recognize what you need." I took that as a huge step in the right direction for myself. In the past, I was either only focused on myself and pursuing what I thought I needed or I was so busy considering everyone else's needs that I was unable to even know my own. When I was focused on myself, I was at my loneliest, and when

I only cared for others, I was the most exhausted and became bitter. God does not want us to live in either state.

Nurturing our spiritual well-being is essential to caring for our whole selves. With Jesus' guidance, we are able to better understand how to care for ourselves. Faith is the foundation of the Church, and He calls us to rely on that same faith as our cornerstone. The Bible tells us that "faith is the realization of what is hoped for and evidence of things not seen" (Hebrews 11:1). We hope for eternity in heaven, and God provides evidence through the life, death, and Resurrection of Jesus.

In This World, There Will Be Suffering

The "fourth trimester," the first three months after birth, is a season unlike any other. It is a sacred and tender time, when the bond between mother and child deepens through every sleepless night and quiet feeding. But it is also a time marked by profound physical, emotional, and spiritual upheaval.

Much of the world romanticizes this stage. Picture-perfect images of swaddled newborns and glowing mothers often fill social media and parenting books. Friends and family may comment, "Cherish every moment," or "These are the best days." Yet beneath the surface, many mothers find themselves suffering in silence, feeling that their struggles are somehow out of step with what's expected.

Physically, the body is in recovery. Whether the birth was smooth or complicated, the process leaves both seen and unseen wounds. Soreness, bleeding, stitches, or surgical healing can make basic movements difficult. Breastfeeding, though beautiful, can be painful and discouraging in the early days. And amid all this, rest is nearly impossible. Newborns wake often, and sleep comes in broken fragments, if at all.

Emotionally, the fourth trimester can feel like a storm. Hormones shift dramatically, tears may fall without explanation, and even joyful moments can feel overwhelming. A new mother may question her identity, wondering who she is now, or she may grieve the loss of life as it once was. There may be feelings of guilt or shame for not loving every moment, or for needing help. Postpartum depression and anxiety are common but still shrouded in stigma, making it hard to speak honestly, even to close friends or within the Church.

NICOLE'S EXPERIENCE WITH POSTPARTUM DEPRESSION

Praise God that postpartum depression, anxiety, and mental illness are more acceptable topics to discuss than in the past. However, this acceptance often fades when we ourselves are the ones suffering. Especially for individuals in caring professions, struggling with a diagnosis can seem like falling short.

During the last trimester of my first pregnancy, I told my OBGYN about my grandmother's struggle with severe bipolar disorder beginning with the birth of her firstborn. My doctor kindly understood the story as code for being concerned for myself and wanting to have a small threshold for starting medications. Two weeks after Evan's birth, I held my baby tightly in my arms, crying uncontrollably. The intense feelings of despair, despite my utter joy as a new mom, were more than I could bear. Worst of all, I believed the lie that I was not good enough to be a mom, especially not to a perfectly healthy and beautiful baby boy.

Fortunately, I knew to communicate my feelings with my doctor, who quickly prescribed treatment. The antidepression medication took time to work, but fortunately family and friends were there to provide love and reassurance. I started counseling, hoping to eventually stop the medication. In my heart, I knew recovery would be a long process, but I refused to accept it. Instead, I denied the possibility that I might have anything resembling my grandmother's mental illness. I convinced myself this was just temporary. Yet each time I considered stopping the medication, life's challenges forced me not only to continue but sometimes to increase the dose.

"But he said to me, 'My grace is sufficient for you, for my power is made perfect in weakness.' I will all the more gladly boast of my weaknesses, that the power of Christ may rest upon me."

—2 Corinthians 12:9

Some well-intended friends told me I needed to pray more, while others said to wait for the hormones to balance and keep breastfeeding. Although these suggestions had merit, the advice sent me into more of a downward spiral. Satan's lies grew stronger: that I wasn't good enough, that I just needed to try harder to overcome depression. An inexplicable anger made me feel like climbing out of my skin, and I feared saying something that might damage my family relationships. I struggled with a despair that made no sense given my many blessings. In my search for relief, I alternated between trying to control everything and sleeping to escape. These overwhelming thoughts and emotions consumed me. I had to claim my weaknesses and allow Christ's power to show me the way to health.

All aspects of my health were in desperate need of attention. As I sought help for my mental health, I quickly realized my spiritual health was also suffering. Through prayer and counseling, God revealed how His presence connects and sustains every part of our being. Though I felt broken, His grace offered restoration. I wanted to be whole again—to become the mother He created me to be. As I allowed God to strengthen my foundation of faith, I recognized my need for ongoing help with depression and anxiety. The more I embraced His healing presence, the more I could seek, find, and receive the help I needed. My spiritual renewal naturally led to improvements in my mental and physical health as well.

Mental illness can affect anyone; it is not a sign of weak faith or personal failure. Like any medical condition, it requires professional treatment and holistic care. We don't tell people with heart disease to pray more; we guide them to see a cardiologist while supporting them spiritually. God works through both prayer and medicine, and following His guidance often means accepting the help He provides through healthcare professionals.

The graces I received were the love of friends and family, the doctor listening to my symptoms and starting medication, finding the right therapist, and eventually accepting the way God made me. By God's grace, I am well today and able to speak openly about this aspect of my life. I pray that you will recognize any and all weaknesses as an opportunity for God to reveal the amazing graces he wishes to bestow on you. For those who have not experienced postpartum depression, showing compassion and support to your sisters who are struggling can help break the silence and shame.

Spiritually, this time can feel disorienting. Time for prayer may disappear. Participation in the sacraments may feel difficult or impossible. A once-strong faith may feel distant. And yet this, too, can be part of our hidden crosses—a purifying fire through which we are invited into deeper union with Christ.

Many people, even well-meaning ones, may fail to recognize the full weight of this season. The world often expects quick recovery, cheerful gratitude, and effortless motherhood. When we express our struggles, we may be met with discomfort, redirection, or advice instead of listening. This response, though subtle, can compound the pain and leave us feeling unseen or dismissed.

Within the Church, there is room for honesty. Scripture does not shy away from lament. Christ Himself wept, grew weary, and asked for help. The saints were no strangers to suffering, and Our Lady, in her quiet strength, carried the full weight of maternal sorrow and joy. God's heart makes space for the entire truth of the postpartum season, embracing both its beauty and its crosses.

The early stages of infancy are a period of immense transformation as you navigate the beautiful yet challenging journey into motherhood. Each day and night brings new experiences that reshape your identity and deepen your faith. While the world may not always recognize the real challenges of this season, Christ walks closely with you, present in every hidden sacrifice and whispered prayer. In those quiet moments, He gently reminds you: *You are not alone. I am with you always.*

In the Catholic faith, suffering holds profound significance, and understanding how to unite our suffering to Christ's sacrifice can provide solace, strength, and purpose in the midst of life's trials. Suffering is not something to be avoided or dismissed, but rather an opportunity for growth, redemption, and deeper communion with

Christ. Through His suffering on the Cross, Jesus transformed pain into an act of perfect love for all humanity. He gave us a model of redemptive suffering that allows even our most difficult moments to be filled with grace.

St. Paul beautifully captures this in Colossians 1:24: "Now I rejoice in my sufferings for your sake, and in my flesh I am filling up what is lacking in the afflictions of Christ on behalf of his body, which is the Church." This teaching reminds us that nothing is wasted when it is offered with love.

For new mothers, this is especially meaningful. The sleepless nights, the aching body, and the emotional weight can all become acts of sacrificial love. Every feeding, every diaper changed, every tear wiped away becomes an expression of Christ's love. In choosing to give oneself for the sake of another, we can mirror Christ's own self-gift for the salvation of the world.

And just as Christ experienced sorrow and anguish, so too can we find comfort in knowing He understands every emotional high and low. In the Garden of Gethsemane, He cried out in distress: "My Father, if it is possible, let this cup pass from me; yet not as I will, but as you will" (Matthew 26:39). He did not shy away from the pain but embraced it with trust in the Father. In moments when we feel weak and overwhelmed, Christ is near, offering both compassion and support.

Uniting your suffering to Christ's brings spiritual fruit not only in your own heart, but also in the lives of others. Every act of surrender, when joined to the Cross, becomes a channel of grace. It can be offered for your child, your spouse, your community, or even the wider world. This spiritual offering becomes a powerful prayer of love and intercession. St. John Paul II wrote:

> Suffering is present in the world in order to release love, in order to give birth to works of love toward neighbor, in order to transform the whole of human civilization into a "civilization of love."[52]

These words hold special meaning for mothers, whose daily sacrifices lay the foundation for that civilization of love, beginning in the home and radiating outward.

Embracing suffering does not mean carrying it alone, however. The beauty of the Catholic faith lies in its communion of saints, believers, and shared burdens. Christ bears the weight alongside each mother, and the Church can provide real help and support. Reach out to other mothers, trusted friends, your parish, or a spiritual advisor. Let them remind you that you belong to the body of Christ, where we uphold and strengthen one another through grace.

Motherhood is a vocation that leads us to grow in faith. In uniting suffering with Christ, this journey becomes not only one of survival, but of transformation. Every trial becomes a path to deeper holiness. Every sacrifice, when offered with love, deepens our relationship with Christ.

You are not alone. In Christ, suffering becomes redemptive. In the Church, it becomes shared. And in the heart of a mother, it becomes a holy offering that echoes through eternity.

Acknowledging the hard things doesn't take away from the love; instead, it creates space for healing. In the midst of it all, you are not alone. There is strength in your surrender, courage in your care, and sacredness in simply showing up each day.

In Chapter 5 of Mark's Gospel, the story of the woman with the hemorrhage reveals the depth of God's unwavering compassion

---

52   John Paul II, *Salvifici Doloris*, sec. VII, February 11, 1984, vatican.va, https://www.vatican.va/content/john-paul-ii/en/apost_letters/1984/documents/hf_jp-ii_apl_11021984_salvifici-doloris.html.

and care. For twelve long years, she suffered physically, was cut off from her community, spent all she had on failed treatments, and was left utterly alone. Considered unclean under the law, she had been told that she was unworthy, that she didn't belong, and that she should stay hidden. And yet, in the midst of her suffering and isolation, she made a bold, faith-filled decision: She leaned in. She reached for Jesus despite the voices around her, the rules, the fear, and the shame. Believing that even touching the hem of His cloak could bring healing, she pressed through the crowd and stretched out her hand. And it did bring healing. Her courageous act of faith did not go unnoticed. Jesus not only restored her health but also acknowledged her dignity, calling her "daughter" and affirming her publicly (see Mark 5:25–34).

This powerful encounter reminds us that no suffering goes unseen by God. His love reaches into the deepest places of our pain, embracing the brokenhearted and the marginalized. Like the hemorrhaging woman, we too are invited to press in, to lean on Christ in our weakness and uncertainty. God does not turn away from our need; He waits patiently for us to turn to Him. He longs for us to reach out in faith, no matter how fragile, even when others or our own inner voice try to convince us we are not worthy. When we do, He meets us with healing, grace, and love. When we lean into Him, we find not only restoration, but also the assurance that we are never alone. We are deeply known, cherished, and held in the heart of our Savior.

This woman's story is also a beautiful call to holistic self-care. She did not passively accept her suffering or resign herself to despair. Instead, she took action to pursue healing. In her act of reaching for Jesus, she cared for her body, soul, and spirit. Likewise, we are called to care for ourselves in a way that reflects our dignity as beloved children of God. Tending to our physical needs, acknowledging our emotional wounds, and seeking spiritual renewal are not selfish acts; they are sacred ones.

Like the hemorrhaging woman, we are invited to approach Christ in faith, trusting that He desires to restore us completely.

Self-Care

Prioritizing self-care is essential for maintaining your mental and physical health while navigating the demands of motherhood. Taking care of yourself allows you to be a better caregiver to your children and promotes overall well-being. The importance of sleep, physical activity, and healthy eating have been discussed earlier in the book. Here are some additional ideas to help you incorporate self-care:

- **Make time for yourself:** Carve out moments of solitude to recharge. Even just a few minutes can have positive benefits. If your baby enjoys a ride, a walk or drive can be helpful!

- **Connect with others:** Socialize with friends or join local mom groups to share experiences and support. Connecting with others who understand the challenges of motherhood can be uplifting and provide a sense of belonging. Promoting healthy relationships is an effective way to create a network of love and support that uplifts your spirit.

- **Practice mindfulness:** Incorporate mindfulness or meditation into your day. Taking a few minutes to focus on your breathing and clear your mind can reduce stress and improve your ability to handle challenging situations.

- **Limit screen time:** Reduce excessive screen time, especially on social media. Remember that people often share their highlight reels, not the full picture. Comparing yourself to others can lead to unnecessary stress and unrealistic expectations. Focus on your journey and celebrate your accomplishments.

- **Talk about your feelings:** Openly communicate with your spouse or a close friend about your feelings and struggles. Bottling up emotions can be detrimental to your mental health, while sharing them can provide relief and understanding.

- **Practice self-compassion:** Be kind and compassionate to yourself. Avoid self-criticism and negative self-talk. Treat yourself with the same understanding and empathy you would offer a friend. Embrace self-compassion as an essential aspect of self-care.

- **Celebrate small wins:** Acknowledge and celebrate your achievements, no matter how small they may seem. Being a mother is challenging, and each triumph deserves recognition.

- **Express gratitude:** Cultivate a habit of expressing gratitude for the people in your life. Let them know how much you appreciate and love them. Gratitude promotes positive feelings and strengthens your bonds.

If you are following these tips and still find yourself overwhelmed or struggling with mental health, do not hesitate to seek professional support. Speaking to a therapist or counselor can offer valuable insights and coping strategies.

Mommy Guilt

The first time I heard a friend say, "I have mommy guilt," I felt such relief. *Finally* someone had put words to what I had been feeling. I was constantly trying to live up to my own expectations of perfection and the pressure of what I thought others expected of me. It was exhausting and often sent my thoughts spiraling into an unhealthy place. But thankfully, the Holy Spirit gently reminded me that those thoughts were not rooted in truth; they were lies. Each day, He invites us to refocus on what is true. Jesus said, "I came so that they might have life and have it more abundantly" (John 10:10).

When the enemy tries to weigh us down with the "should haves" of motherhood and life, we can pray for the grace to remember God's truth: His presence, His mercy, and His guidance.

It's important to acknowledge our feelings without judgment. Mommy guilt is real, but it does not define us. Parenting is full of hard decisions, and it's natural to feel unsure at times. When guilt creeps in, we can pause and identify where it is coming from. Is it societal pressure? Comparison? Unrealistic expectations? Understanding the source helps us to bring those feelings into the open and deal with them with grace.

In my sixteen years as a mom, I've worked full-time, part-time, and even stayed home for a season. I can honestly say that the hardest season was being home full-time. But no matter the role, there is always some level of sacrifice. And yet, through it all, the call remains the same: to bring our children to the Lord. That calling will look different in every family and every season, and that's okay. There is no blueprint for perfect parenting, because perfection does not exist in this world. What does exist is God's abundant grace and mercy, ready for us every day.

We can challenge the negative thoughts that tell us we are not enough or that we are doing it all wrong. Instead, we can focus on the truth: We are deeply loved, and God is walking with us. Let's set realistic expectations, give ourselves permission to make mistakes, and focus not on the quantity of time we spend with our children, but on the quality. When we are present and intentional, those moments matter more than we often realize.

During Mass recently, I was moved by the song "Change Our Hearts" by Rory Cooney. The reminder that earth is not our ultimate home is a beautiful promise and difficult to comprehend. It reminded me that this life is not heaven. We will be pulled between joy and struggle, hope and disappointment. But God is always inviting us closer, calling us to say *yes* to His voice, to lean in to Jesus, and to let Him lead us.

So, at the end of each day as we pray, we can ask God to guide our reflection. We can thank Him for whatever the day held and ask for His peace to settle over our hearts. There is no need for guilt when we have His grace. Let's choose to walk in that truth and allow Him to shape us as mothers, women, and beloved daughters of the King.

Being while Doing

In a recent conversation with my sister, we were reflecting on the tension we so often feel between *doing* and *being*. It's a paradox we live in as mothers and as followers of Christ. On one hand, we are encouraged to be present—to live in the moment, be still, be available, and engaged with those around us. On the other hand, our days are filled with endless tasks—changing diapers, doing the laundry, washing dishes, preparing meals. The *doing* never stops.

This tension reflects the deeper reality of our lives as women walking the path between heaven and earth. We are called to carry our cross daily, to walk this earthly journey with our eyes and hearts set on eternal things. Scripture tells us to "pray always," and yet, we live in the mess and the noise of everyday life. This creates friction, an internal push-and-pull that can be overwhelming if we try to carry it alone.

But we were never meant to walk this road without nourishment. We are given the gift of the Eucharist, which is spiritual nourishment from Christ Himself. And we are meant to be encouraged and supported by our brothers and sisters in Christ. Every time we come to the altar, we say, "Lord, I am not worthy"—and it's true that, on our own, we are not. Yet we are made worthy not by what we do, but by the sacrifice of Jesus. Through His Death and Resurrection, He calls us His beloved. He calls us His friends. He no longer sees us as slaves but as daughters and sons. This identity is the foundation for how we live, how we love, and how we mother.

The real issue goes beyond doing versus being. It is *how we are being while we are doing*. These are not separate paths; we are called to practice both. God has given us the task of stewarding this life. He calls us to serve, to love, to act. He gives us work to do with our hands and hearts. But even as we do, we are invited to *be*: to be rooted in Him, to be present, to be a conduit of His Spirit.

As a new mother, your world centers around caring for your infant, your family, and yourself. These are sacred callings. You may hear countless opinions on what you *should* be doing, but your focus should remain on what truly matters: your relationship with your Heavenly Father, your health and wholeness, your baby's well-being, and the peace of your home. Everything else is secondary.

And as you do all these things, whether it is rocking your baby at 3:00 a.m. or folding a mountain of laundry, remember this: You are not just doing it *for* God; you are doing it *with* Him. You are a beloved daughter, beautifully and wonderfully made, and through you, the love of Jesus flows into your home. You are the hands of Christ. You are His presence in your child's life. So be gentle with yourself. Be present. And let the *being* and the *doing* become one beautiful, holy offering.

In Summary

As we have explored throughout this chapter, motherhood is a beautiful, challenging journey that requires you to take care of yourself in addition to your infant. This might mean taking a few minutes to pray while your baby naps, accepting help from those who offer to bring meals, or simply allowing yourself grace when the laundry sits unfolded for another day. Remember, dear sisters, your worth is not measured by the number of tasks you complete or how clean your home is but by the love you pour into your children and yourself.

God's grace meets you exactly where you are: during the sleepless nights, moments of doubt, physical recovery, and emotional highs and lows. He sees your struggles, your sacrifices, and your heart. As Psalm 73:26 states: *"Though my flesh and my heart fail, God is the rock of my heart, my portion forever."*

Remember, in the midst of suffering, fatigue, or feeling overwhelmed, God is always there for you. He deeply cares for you and loves you unconditionally. Your journey of motherhood is unique; no two days are the same. Some days you may feel like you are barely hanging on, and other days will overflow with joy and wonder. In both seasons, God's love remains constant. When that voice in your head says you are not enough, His grace gently reminds you that you are. Motherhood is a beautiful yet challenging path, but you never walk it alone. God's presence surrounds you, offering strength in weariness, comfort in sorrow, and unwavering guidance as you live out this sacred calling.

Take heart. You are doing holy work. Embrace grace. Extend compassion to yourself. Trust in God's plan. You are exactly the mother your child needs.

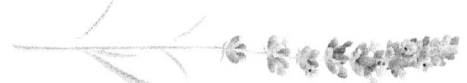

READ: *"May the God of hope fill you with all joy and peace in believing, so that you may abound in hope by the power of the holy Spirit."* (Romans 15:13)

MEDITATE: Gaze upon a crucifix, holy image of the sacred heart of Jesus, or other meaningful art as you pray or listen to music.

PRAY: Let nothing disturb you,
Let nothing frighten you,
All things are passing away:
God never changes.
Patience obtains all things
Whoever has God lacks nothing;
God alone suffices. —St. Teresa of Avila

LISTEN: "Meet Me at the Well" by Regnum Christi

RESOLVE

1. What is one step that you can take to promote your self-care?
2. How can you invite Christ into your suffering and allow His grace to restore you?

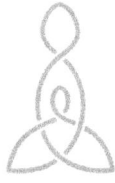

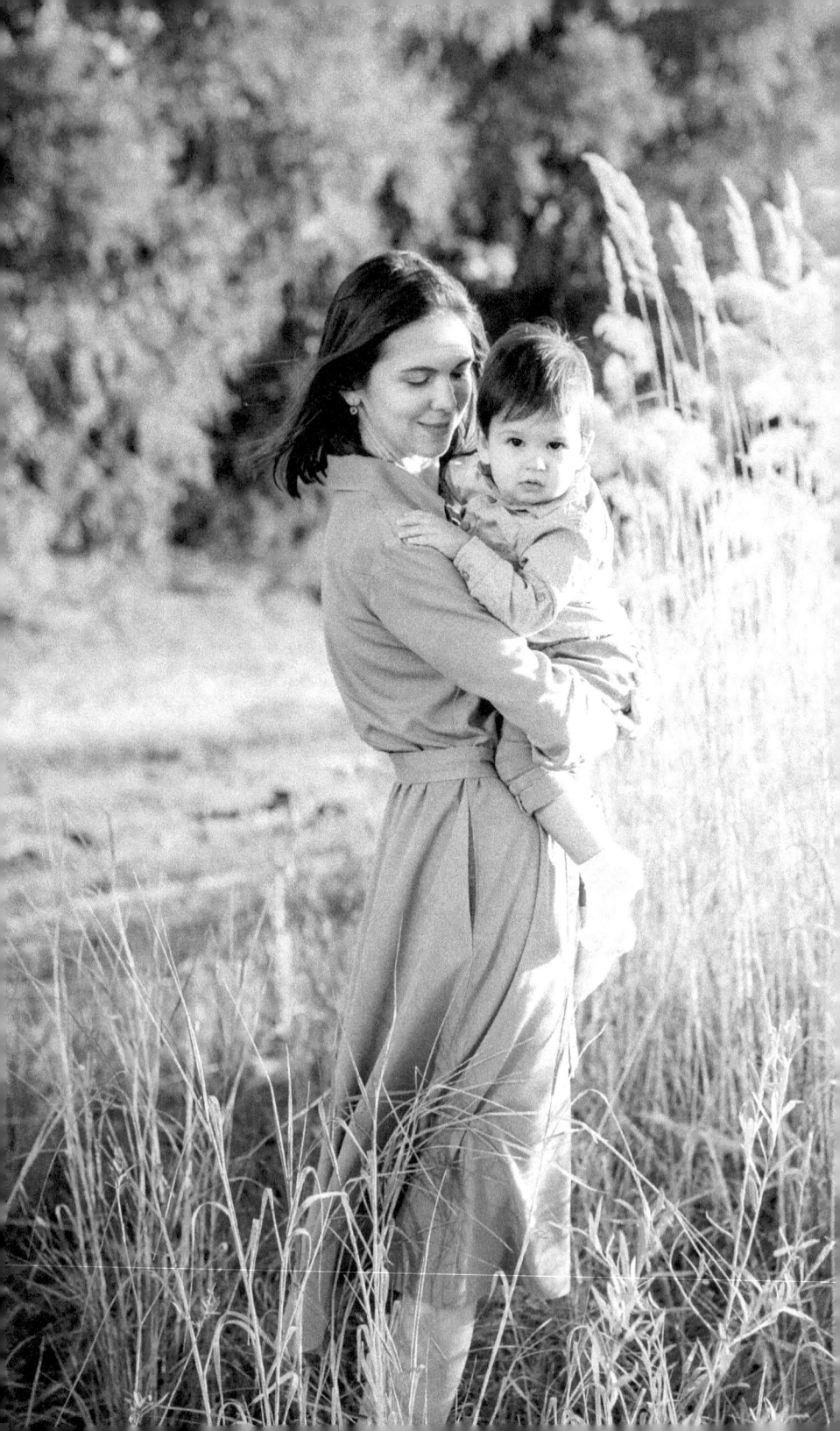

CHAPTER 12

Finding Calm in the Storm

"He woke up, rebuked the wind, and said to the sea, "Quiet!
Be still!" The wind ceased and there was great calm."

—Mark 4:39

About two weeks before I was to return to work after maternity leave and a day before my older son's eighth birthday, Hurricane Harvey hit Houston with a vengeance. The four days of nonstop rain brought Houston approximately fifty inches of precipitation, about the same amount that falls in a one-year period! As we played board games in the living room to distract ourselves, my husband and I realized we needed to plan for the worst. Seemingly far-fetched conversations about kayaks, waders, and infant carriers became serious. As the water approached the back door, the neighborhood men cleared the street drains of debris at all hours of the night. At home, I comforted our children and prayed mightily for our safety. The story of Jesus rebuking the wind and sea came to mind and by some miracle, we were able to get a bit of sleep.

Family and friends called to check on us and ask if they could help in any way. Our answer was always the same: "Please pray!" When the skies cleared and the water in the backyard receded, we gratefully reported that water never came into our home! We were safe, dry, and relieved.

Jesus Is in the Boat with Us in the Midst of the Storm

Life has a way of showing us how little control we truly have. During the storm, I found myself feeling overwhelmed by fear and uncertainty. A sense of helplessness was looming, but we knew we needed to stay focused on God's love and ever-present support. It was exactly during those moments that God's grace showed up! Despite the rain, wind, and rising waters, we were able to find serenity in the situation. Looking back, we are able to even see some humor! My oldest son still remembers celebrating his birthday in the living room, being allowed to watch endless movies on DVD—thank goodness we kept those around! My husband and I also grew closer as we pulled together to create an optimistic and hopeful environment for our children.

It is during these distressing moments that Jesus Christ stands as a sign of hope, offering comfort and peace amidst the storm. As the epitome of love and compassion, Jesus serves as the ultimate source of solace and peace. He alone can provide us with the strength and reassurance we need to navigate through such challenging times. He doesn't promise to remove our struggles or to calm the storms in our lives, but He does promise to be a constant source of hope and tranquility.

When the disciples in the boat found Jesus sleeping, they asked Him if He even cared (Mark 4:38). The truth is that He sees us in our struggles and He cares deeply.

Jesus' teachings emphasize the power of faith and prayer. When we are facing the distress of sickness, turning to Jesus in prayer becomes a means of finding peace and acceptance. Trusting in His divine plan, we can relinquish our fears and worries, finding strength in the knowledge that we and our children are held in the loving hands of the Savior.

Jesus' calming presence during storms, as depicted in the biblical narrative of calming the storm on the Sea of Galilee, is a perfect example of his unwavering support. Jesus can bring the same peace to our turbulent or anxious hearts. Know that He is always available to you and wants you to call upon Him. "When he disembarked and saw the vast crowd, his heart was moved with pity for them and he cured their sick" (Matthew 14:14).

Once we knew we were in the clear from the water coming into our home, we breathed a sigh of relief. However, just as we thought the storm had passed, we faced another crisis. The flood's aftermath brought airborne irritants that triggered respiratory problems across the city, and our two-month-old baby Charlie fell ill. In the middle of the night, Charlie's breathing became rapid and labored, with visible strain in the muscles of his ribcage and flaring nostrils. Despite our best efforts with nasal saline and fever medication, his condition worsened.

The situation felt especially dire because emergency services had been suspended and a citywide curfew was in effect. Yet as a new sense of helplessness threatened to overwhelm us, we felt God's presence guiding our decisions. My mommy intuition knew we needed to do something more than stay home. I said a prayer for guidance and knew that we needed to drive to the children's hospital emergency room. Driving on the nearly empty interstate, we didn't feel alone or abandoned. We prayed during the drive and knew we were going to be okay.

Upon arrival at the ER, Charlie's oxygen saturation was 89 percent, well below the normal range. But just as Jesus calmed the stormy seas, He calmed our fears. After nebulizer treatments, Charlie's breathing normalized and his oxygen levels rose to 97 percent. After being monitored for a couple of hours, we were told he had a respiratory virus but we could take him home. Praise be to God, breathing treatments and fever medications were all he needed. Driving home, my husband and I marveled at the surreal peace we'd felt throughout the ordeal. Though the situation was serious, our trust in God had kept panic at bay, allowing us to focus clearly on Charlie's needs.

Throughout Scripture, we see how Jesus meets people exactly where they are, providing exactly what they need: physical healing, emotional comfort, and spiritual guidance. In our own moments of worry, we can trust in His unchanging nature. Jesus is present and walks alongside us through every challenge we face as parents.

When I find myself anxious over my children having some kind of an illness, I am reminded of our Mother Mary and how she must have felt whenever she had to face difficult challenges raising Jesus. The first one that we hear about is when she and Joseph bring Jesus to the temple, where Simeon tells her "you yourself a sword will pierce" (Luke 2:35). Can you imagine what it must have felt like to be a new mom and hear someone tell you this? But Mary leaned on God and His almighty power and grace and knew her ultimate goal was to do God's will.

Another time we hear of a challenge Mary faced is when she couldn't find Jesus after they had traveled to Jerusalem for Passover when Jesus was twelve years old. Mary and Joseph searched for Jesus for three days before finding him! Mary tells Jesus that she had "great anxiety" over his absence, and Jesus's response was, "Why were you looking for me? Did you not know that I must be in my Father's house?" After they returned to Nazareth, we are told that Mary "kept all these things in her heart" (Luke 2:41–51).

To do God's will means we accept that His way may not be ours. The storms of life are most certainly not something that we expect or want. Sometimes the storms are large events in our society that impact all those around us. Sometimes, however, the storms are seemingly insignificant to others but impactful to our own mental or physical well-being. God asks that we accept His will and lean in and do as Mary did. When Gabriel came to Mary and announced that she had been chosen by God to carry Jesus in her womb, we know "she was greatly troubled at what was said and pondered what sort of greeting this might be" (Luke 1:29). Yet she was still able to respond to Gabriel with these words: "May it be done to me according to your word" (Luke 1:38). During times of trial, anxiety, or uncertainty, may we turn to God as Mary did and accept His way. We can have assurance that through all the storms, He will not leave us. He will guide us and keep us ever close to Him.

Encountering illness and sickness is an inevitable aspect of raising children. Differentiating between minor illnesses, those requiring primary care, those needing urgent care, and those demanding ER attention empowers us to provide the appropriate level of medical attention. While some illnesses can be managed at home with home care and over-the-counter medications, others may require evaluation by a primary care physician or an urgent care facility. In life-threatening situations, seeking immediate medical attention at the ER is critical. Being informed and prepared allows us to navigate these challenging moments with confidence, ensuring the health and well-being of our beloved children.

When to Seek Help

The most frequent time medical advice is sought is in the midst of an illness or acute injury. Knowing your baby's baseline behavior and typical way of being is extremely helpful. On numerous occasions, parents brought their child to the clinic where I worked and simply stated, "They are just acting differently." Changes can include atypical feeding or sleeping patterns, different bowel movements or urination habits, or change in activity or personality (such as increased irritability).

While many childhood illnesses and injuries can be managed at home or with a visit to the pediatrician, sometimes it's challenging to determine whether a visit to the office, an urgent care, or the emergency room is necessary. If you are in doubt about whether you should take your infant to see a medical provider, call their office first. Pediatric offices should have an on-call provider or triage nurse available to answer questions and help you determine what kind of care your child requires. A pediatric healthcare provider can talk you through your observations or concerns and identify if a treatment plan is indicated. Remember, not all illnesses or injuries may need intervention.

While there are many medical care options available today, remember that your pediatric provider knows your child and their history best, and if it is feasible and not an emergency, they are the most qualified to evaluate your infant. Not all urgent care facilities or telehealth providers may be comfortable seeing young infants, and sometimes treatments for adults are different from those recommended for young children.

Though your pediatric provider's office is the preferred medical home for your infant, there are certain situations that require immediate medical attention. Here are ten common reasons it's time to take a child to the emergency department:

1. **Difficulty breathing:** If a child is having severe difficulty breathing, such as gasping for air, noisy breathing, or showing signs of respiratory distress, seek immediate medical attention.

2. **Severe allergic reaction:** Symptoms like difficulty breathing, swelling of the face or throat, hives, repetitive vomiting, or change in level of awareness may be signs of anaphylaxis (a potentially life-threatening reaction). If you suspect a severe allergic reaction, go to the ER immediately. Administering epinephrine (if already prescribed) and seeking immediate medical help is essential in these situations.

3. **Head injury:** Any head injury that involves loss of consciousness, confusion, persistent vomiting, seizures, or a significant change in behavior requires immediate medical evaluation. These symptoms may indicate a more serious head injury and require prompt medical attention.

4. **Persistent fever or fever with concerning symptoms:** Any fever in newborns (under three months old) should be evaluated urgently whether or not they have other symptoms and regardless of how long the fever has lasted. If an older infant's fever is persistent or accompanied by symptoms like a change in appetite, decreased wet diapers, persistent vomiting, lethargy, or irritability, seek medical attention.

5. **Seizures:** Any seizure in an infant is scary and deserves medical attention. If your child has a first time seizure, they should be evaluated by a medical provider. If a child experiences a seizure that lasts longer than five minutes, or they have multiple seizures in a row without fully regaining consciousness, it is a medical emergency, and you should call 911.

6. **Severe dehydration:** Signs of severe dehydration in a child include sunken eyes, dry mouth, lack of tears, lethargy, unsteadiness, or decreased urine output. Even if they are keeping some fluids down, if they have signs of severe dehydration, your child should be evaluated.

7. **Severe abdominal pain:** Intense or persistent abdominal pain, especially if it is accompanied by fever, vomiting, or blood in the stool, requires medical attention.

8. **Suspected broken bones:** Broken bones in infants are not as common as they are in older children, but they can occur at times. If an infant has a suspected fracture or significant injury, such as a limb that appears deformed, an inability to move a body part, or severe pain, go to the emergency department for assessment, imaging, and appropriate treatment.

9. **Severe burns:** Burns that are large, deep, involve sensitive skin areas, or are caused by chemicals or electricity require immediate medical attention.

10. **Ingestion of toxic substances:** If a child ingests a toxic substance, such as medication, cleaning products, or household chemicals, contact a poison control center or go to the emergency department immediately.

This is not an exhaustive list, and if you are ever unsure or concerned about a child's health or well-being, it's always better to err on the side of caution and seek medical advice.

In Summary

As mothers, we will inevitably face storms and times when life feels overwhelming, uncertain, and beyond our control. But in these moments, we are not alone. Just as Jesus calmed the storm for His disciples, He promises to calm the storms in our hearts as well. Jesus told us, "Peace I leave with you; my peace I give to you. Not as the world gives do I give it to you. Do not let your hearts be troubled or afraid" (John 14:27).

When storms come, remember that seeking help is not a sign of weakness but an act of wisdom. Whether it's reaching out to a friend, a healthcare professional, or God Himself, there is no shame in acknowledging that we can't do it all alone. The moments when we are called to seek help are opportunities for growth, for surrendering our need to control, and for trusting that God has us and our babies in His hands.

As you navigate the ups and downs of motherhood, remember that the storms will pass. You will weather them, and you will come out stronger. When the waves of fear and uncertainty seem too high, take comfort in knowing that Jesus is in the boat with you, offering peace. And as you walk in the footsteps of Mary, find courage in her example: a mother who loved, trusted, and stayed, no matter what the storm brought. You are never alone, and you are never without hope.

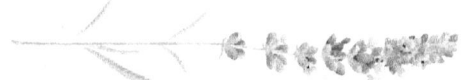

READ: *"I have told you this so that you might have peace in me. In the world you will have trouble, but take courage, I have conquered the world."* (John 16:33)

MEDITATE: Remember the song "Mary Had a Little Lamb"? This may seem like a simple rhyme, but through a Christian lens, it reflects the peace of Christ. Mary, the mother of Jesus, carried the Lamb of God—pure and full of love. Just as the lamb followed Mary closely, Jesus stays near to us, bringing peace to our homes and hearts.

PRAY: God, grant me the serenity to accept the things I cannot change, the courage to change the things I can, and the wisdom to know the difference. —Serenity Prayer

LISTEN: "Peace Be Still" by Hope Darst

RESOLVE

1. The next time you encounter stress, no matter how small or large, say the Serenity Prayer.
2. Sing "Mary had a Little Lamb" to your baby and tell them of the pure lamb of God and His love.

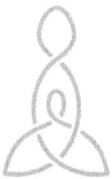

CHAPTER 13

Helping Your Baby Thrive!

"For you were called for freedom, brothers.
But do not use this freedom as an opportunity for the flesh;
rather, serve one another through love."

—Galatians 5:13

My husband and I are part of a marriage ministry called Teams of Our Lady. We get together once a month to share a meal, read Scripture, pray together, and encourage one another in our vocations of marriage. One of the essential tenets is to have a "Rule of Life." This rule is intended to provide a common ground for the family to constantly return to for guidance. St. Paul's letter to the Galatians serves as the verse from which we wrote our "Rule of Life."

Use Your Freedom to Love and Shine

In his letter to the Galatian church, the Apostle Paul emphasizes the importance of living a life guided by love and the Holy Spirit. St. Paul presents a powerful explanation about how genuine freedom should be expressed through love. As believers, we are called to embrace the freedom that comes from faith in Christ and the indwelling of the Holy Spirit. True freedom is an opportunity to choose a life that expresses love and care for others. Living out this freedom allows us to embrace Christ's promise of abundant life. Throughout our Catholic history, saints have demonstrated how to live out their faith by using their freedom to love and serve others. A saint dear to us is St. Gianna Molla.

From a young age, St. Gianna Beretta Molla was taught to seek Jesus in the faces of those around her. Her parents instilled in her the practice of daily prayer and the importance of recognizing Christ in her neighbors. This foundation shaped her into a woman of deep faith and compassion, a faith she expressed through charitable action and service to others.

Gianna became a pediatrician and dedicated her career to caring for mothers and children. She opened an outpatient health center, offering her expertise and kindness to those in need. Although she once dreamed of serving as a medical missionary, her own chronic health conditions kept her close to home. Through prayer and discernment, she came to understand that her vocation was not only in medicine but also in marriage and motherhood.

Throughout her life, Gianna sought strength and guidance in the sacraments, frequently attending Mass and spending time in Eucharistic adoration. She embraced her daily responsibilities as acts of love, offering every moment to the Lord. She married Pietro Molla, and together they built a family rooted in faith, welcoming four children into the world. Tragically, she also experienced the pain of two miscarriages, yet she remained steadfast in her trust in God's plan.

Gianna's faith was put to the ultimate test when she was diagnosed with a uterine tumor while pregnant with her fourth child. Presented with the option of a hysterectomy, which would have ended her pregnancy, she instead chose a riskier path and underwent surgery to remove the tumor while preserving her unborn child's life. She carried her baby to term and successfully delivered her daughter, Gianna Emanuela. However, severe complications arose shortly after childbirth, and a week later, Gianna passed away, having sacrificed her life for her child's.

St. Gianna's ability to make such a profound choice was not born from a single moment of courage, but from a lifetime of growing in virtue, trust, and reliance on God. She had spent years cultivating a deep connection with the Lord, learning to surrender to His divine will. With the freedom given to her by God, she chose to reflect His love through her selfless acts of service, embracing each decision as an opportunity to glorify Him. Her life radiated the fruits of the Holy Spirit, especially through her charity, generosity, and faithfulness. She embodied charity in her unwavering love for her family, patients, and community. Her generosity was evident in the way she gave of herself without hesitation, whether through her medical practice or in her ultimate sacrifice. Her faithfulness to God was steadfast, guiding every step of her journey, from the small daily acts of devotion to the monumental choices that defined her sainthood.

When she was made a saint in 2004, St. Gianna Molla became the first canonized woman physician and professional who was also a "working mom."[53] She is a patron saint for mothers, doctors, and the pro-life movement. Her legacy is not just that she chose life for her child but that she lived a life of faith, love, and service in all aspects of her vocation.

Her words remind us of the foundation of all fruitful action: "The stillness of prayer is the most essential condition for fruitful action.

Before all else, the disciple kneels down."[54] Whether as a working mother or a stay-at-home mom, we are all called to a life of faith, lived out in our own unique vocation. We are also called to nourish the children God has put in our care to develop their whole health and teach them how to use their freedom to let the fruits of the Holy Spirit shine.

St. Gianna's example challenges us to trust deeply in God, serve our families and communities with love, and recognize that even in the ordinary, we are called to holiness. Just as her mother taught her to seek Jesus, we too have the responsibility of guiding those in our care toward sainthood. The next great saint may very well be growing under our roof, and it is through our daily faithfulness that we help shape them into who God created them to be.

Fruits of the Holy Spirit

Just as St. Gianna exhibited fruits of the Holy Spirit, we can reveal the fruit of the Spirit to our own families. These virtues—charity, joy, peace, patience, kindness, goodness, generosity, gentleness, faithfulness, modesty, self-control, and chastity —are the evidence of a life lived in the Spirit (see *CCC*, 1832) and reflect Christ's character. Using our freedom to love means actively choosing to express these fruits in our interactions with others. It involves setting aside our own interests and desires to prioritize the well-being of those around us.

As we journey along the path of motherhood, God calls us to be willing to be transformed to be more like Him. This is only possible by entering a closer relationship with God and asking Him to shape and guide us. The fruits of the Holy Spirit offer concrete ways we can

---

54	Catholic Storeroom, "The Stillness of Prayer: Saint Gianna Beretta Molla," accessed March 25, 2025, https://www.catholicstoreroom.com/2017/02/18/stillness-of-prayer/.

be shaped to live and interact with ourselves, our children, family, and community. As mothers, we can become living testimonies of His grace and transformative power. The following is a brief exploration of how we can embody each fruit:

- **Charity (Love):** We can demonstrate charity and unconditional love by nurturing and caring for our children and spouse. We are first called to love, seeking nothing in return. Charity prioritizes our family's well-being through small acts of service.

- **Joy:** Despite the challenges and demands of motherhood, we can choose joy by finding gratitude in the blessings of our children and the gift of motherhood that has been bestowed on us. We can strive to create a joyful atmosphere at home, fostering an environment of laughter, positivity, and contentment.

- **Peace:** I love hearing the words "May peace be with you." It is my favorite time of the Mass. God truly wants us to have peace with Him. We can seek inner peace through prayer and surrendering our will to God. Forgiveness and open communication are ways to encourage peace.

- **Patience:** Motherhood often tests one's patience! I must admit that I am often reminded to take the advice I give my children when they are becoming impatient. I tell them, "Look at this as a gift from God to practice your patience." Praise God for His infinite mercy and patience with me. I find that truly listening and calming my response serves myself and my family. Prayer and deep breathing contribute significantly to cultivating patience.

- **Kindness:** We can do this by showing compassion, empathy, and generosity to everyone! Small acts of service help to cultivate this virtue.

- **Goodness:** Our words and actions are powerful. We can model honesty and integrity through them. Making choices that prioritize our child's well-being over convenience and teaching ethical behavior through our example show that we want to do God's will.

- **Generosity:** We show generosity when we give freely of our time, resources, and self without reluctance. Sharing our attention fully when our child needs us, even amid competing responsibilities, and giving of ourselves beyond what seems possible are examples of generosity.

- **Gentleness:** This virtue can be lived by offering comfort and a gentle touch and creating a safe and nurturing environment. Guiding with firm but tender correction is another example of being gentle.

- **Faithfulness:** We can exhibit faithfulness by prioritizing our relationship with God. Our children are never too young to be taught the faith. Early and often reading, showing pictures, and attending church establishes a routine and provides consistency. Your baby will grow up with the familiar sights and sounds of a loving God.

- **Modesty:** This describes humility in behavior, appearance, and attitude. Modesty involves a healthy respect for the dignity of the human person and avoiding excessiveness or indecency in both actions and appearance. Modesty is about recognizing the value of our body and how we should treat it (both our own and others) with reverence. It reflects an inner attitude of humility, where we don't seek attention or glory through outward appearances or excessive behaviors. This fruit goes beyond just modest clothing or appearance; it also includes modesty in speech, behavior, and in how we interact socially. We can exhibit modesty by teaching others that worth comes from within rather than external validation.

- **Self-control:** Spending time and energy to understand and manage our changing emotions will serve ourselves and our babies. Responding thoughtfully rather than reactively to challenging behavior, and modeling healthy emotions are examples of practicing self-control. Setting healthy boundaries and practicing self-care in alignment with our values are additional examples.

- **Chastity:** Chastity is the proper integration of human sexuality according to one's state in life, whether single, married, or consecrated. Chastity means living in accordance with God's plan for sexuality, which is always for the good of the person and their relationships. We can demonstrate this fruit by modeling healthy relationships, demonstrating appropriate boundaries, and teaching children to respect their bodies and those of others.

Our lived example will have a lasting impact on our children's lives and reflect the transformative work of the Holy Spirit within them.

Your Baby's Journey toward Holiness

All people are called to holiness; it is a universal invitation from God to embrace a life of righteousness, love, and moral integrity. Seeking holiness involves aligning our hearts with God's will so we may be lights in a broken world. Regardless of background or beliefs, seeking holiness allows us to draw closer to the divine and live lives of purpose and meaning.

As parents, we have a sacred responsibility to guide our young children on the path toward holiness. By fostering a love for God, teaching biblical principles, and living out our faith, we can shape the character and spirituality of our children. Through intentional and consistent efforts, we can help our children develop a strong foundation in faith, enabling them to walk the path of holiness. Each child is fearfully and wonderfully made, bearing the image of the Creator. As we nurture and guide our little ones with love and care, we create an environment for God's light to radiate from within.

Through love and positive affirmation, we foster a sense of security and self-worth in our children. As a result, our child's innate qualities, talents, and gifts can flourish, allowing God's light to shine brightly through their unique personality.

Temperament and Personality: Understanding Your Baby's Unique Traits

As your baby grows, you may observe patterns in the way your baby responds to particular situations. Given these observations, it is helpful to understand infant temperaments and personalities and the differences between them. Temperament refers to the innate traits a baby is born with, which are relatively consistent throughout their life. Personality, on the other hand, develops over time and is shaped by experiences, relationships, and the environment. Understanding a baby's temperament can help you provide care that is better suited to your baby's natural responses.

Researchers have described nine key characteristics that make up a baby's temperament. These traits may help you better understand your baby's natural inclinations and needs:

- **Activity level:** How active or passive your baby is during daily activities

- **Rhythmicity:** The consistency of your baby's biological functions (sleeping, eating, etc.)

- **Approach/withdrawal:** How your baby reacts to new situations or people

- **Adaptability:** How easily your baby adjusts to changes in routine or surroundings

- **Intensity of reaction:** The energy or intensity of your baby's emotional responses

- **Mood:** The general tendency toward a positive or negative mood

- **Persistence/attention span:** How long your baby focuses on an activity or task

- **Distractibility:** How easily your baby is distracted by external stimuli

- **Sensory threshold:** The level of sensitivity to sensory stimuli (light, sound, textures)[55]

Babies often exhibit certain temperament types based on the combination of the above characteristics. Most babies fall into one of three broad categories, though some may show a mix of traits or not fit neatly into any one type. These types are:

- **Easy (or "flexible") baby:** These babies tend to have a predictable and regular routine in terms of sleeping, eating, and mood. They are generally calm, adaptable, and easy to soothe, adjusting well to changes in their environment. Easy babies are typically content.

- **Slow to warm up (or sensitive) baby:** Babies who are sensitive may take longer to adjust to new experiences, people, or changes in their environment. They can be more sensitive to sensory stimuli, becoming easily overwhelmed. While they may need extra comfort and soothing, they typically warm up to new situations over time with gentle encouragement.

---

55   American Academy of Pediatrics, "How to Understand Your Child's Temperament," *HealthyChildren.org*, accessed March 26, 2025, https://www.healthychildren.org/English/ages-stages/gradeschool/Pages/How-to-Understand-Your-Childs-Temperament.aspx.

- **Challenging (or "difficult") baby:** Challenging babies may be more intense in their reactions to stimuli, with a tendency to be irritable or easily upset. They may have irregular sleeping and eating patterns and may resist changes in their routine or environment. These babies often require more patience and effort to soothe and help adjust.[56]

Note that these temperament types are generalizations; each baby is unique. However, understanding these different types can help you provide more personalized care and support in line with your baby's natural responses.

As babies grow and interact with their surroundings, their personality begins to emerge. Unlike temperament, personality traits develop gradually and are influenced by caregiving practices, cultural values, and social interactions. A baby's emerging personality may reflect self-awareness, preferences for certain activities or people, and a developing approach to social interactions. This may be exhibited in behaviors such as being more selective with smiles, vocalizing in response to familiar faces, or showing varying levels of interest in play.

A baby's temperament may also influence their developing personality. For example, a baby who initially displays a challenging temperament may develop a confident or assertive personality over time as they gain more experiences and learn how to navigate the world around them. A baby who is initially more observant and cautious may grow into a thoughtful and social child as they gain confidence in new environments and interactions.

Understanding both temperament and personality can help you offer care that is better suited to your child's unique needs. Recognizing that a baby's temperament is innate and will remain relatively constant allows you to meet your child's needs in ways that align with the way

56   American Academy of Pediatrics, "How to Understand Your Child's Temperament."

God created them. For instance, a slow-to-warm-up baby might need extra time to adjust to new experiences, while an easygoing baby may thrive with more flexibility and spontaneous activities.

At the same time, as your baby's personality develops, you can encourage growth by offering opportunities for social interaction, exploring new activities, and supporting your child's growing sense of self. Paying attention to both your baby's temperament and emerging personality allows you to create an environment that nurtures your child's individual needs and promotes their overall well-being.

Remember, each baby is uniquely created by God, and it may take time and experimentation to discover what techniques work best for your infant. By paying attention to their cues, being patient, and offering love and comfort in ways that respect their temperament and support the development of their personality, you will be helping your baby thrive in a nurturing and soothing environment.

Nurturing Your Baby's Whole Development

Just as we seek to cultivate the fruits of the Spirit in our own lives, we can nurture our baby's development in ways that honor both their physical and spiritual needs. The first twelve months of life represent an extraordinary period of growth in every dimension—physical, cognitive, emotional, and spiritual. The support, care, and nurturing provided by parents and caregivers during this crucial phase play an essential role in fostering healthy growth and setting the stage for a lifetime of development. Below, we will discuss some general suggestions which may help promote healthy development. A detailed list of developmental milestones can be found in Appendix 4.

Responding to your baby goes beyond meeting basic physical needs; it's creating a deep, meaningful connection that forms the basis for their emotional and social development. As a mother, you have an extraordinary opportunity to build a foundation of love, trust, and security through intentional, responsive interactions. Your attentiveness is a sign of your love that helps your baby feel safe, understood, and cherished.

BONDING AND ATTACHMENT

Part of responding to your baby includes engaging in mindful bonding and attachment. This is a crucial and beautiful process that lays the foundation for their emotional and social development. Here are some key points to consider:

- **Skin-to-skin contact:** Holding your baby against your bare skin helps establish a deep connection and promotes feelings of security. It may help regulate your baby's temperature, heart rate, and breathing. It also helps release bonding hormones like oxytocin that benefit both you and your baby.

- **Eye contact and responsive interactions:** Maintaining eye contact with your baby and responding promptly to their cues and needs fosters a sense of trust and connection. Engaging in cooing, talking, and singing encourages communication and promotes attachment.

- **Physical touch and affection:** Regularly cuddling, hugging, and gently stroking or massaging your baby strengthens the bond between you. Physical touch releases feel-good hormones and reinforces a sense of love and security. There is evidence that physical touch promotes bonding and helps brain development in your infant.

- **Feeding time:** Whether breastfeeding or bottle-feeding, feeding your baby offers an intimate bonding experience. Focus on creating a calm and nurturing environment during feedings, making eye contact, and using soft, soothing tones.

- **Baby-wearing and close proximity:** Carrying your baby in a sling or baby carrier allows them to be close to your body, providing comfort and security while allowing you to continue daily activities. The physical proximity fosters a sense of closeness and enhances the bond between you.

Bonding and attachment are built over time through consistent love, care, and responsiveness. Every baby is unique, so be patient and enjoy the process of developing a deep and lasting connection with your little one.

ROCK, TALK, READ, AND PRAY

Responding to your baby through rocking, talking, reading, and praying are also invaluable ways to nurture their development and build a deep connection with them.

Rocking your baby gently in your arms or in a rocking chair provides comfort and security. The rhythmic motion mimics the familiar sensation they experienced in the womb, promoting a sense of calm and relaxation. It also allows for physical closeness, strengthening the bond between you and your little one.

Talking to your baby is a powerful way to engage and stimulate their developing brain. Use a soothing tone and talk about your day, sing lullabies, or simply narrate your activities. This helps build their language skills, enhances their social development, and strengthens the emotional connection between you and your baby.

Reading to your baby, even from a very young age, has numerous benefits. It introduces them to the world of words, stimulates their cognitive development, and fosters a love for books and learning. As you read together, your baby also experiences the comfort of your presence and the soothing sound of your voice.

Praying with your baby is a beautiful way to foster their spiritual growth and establish a sense of faith. It creates a sacred space where you can express gratitude, seek guidance, and pray for your baby's well-being. Praying together instills a sense of connection with God and can bring peace and comfort to both you and your baby.

Responding to your baby in these ways is vital for their emotional, cognitive, and spiritual development. It demonstrates that their needs are seen, heard, and valued, creating a secure attachment between you. Through these interactions, you lay the foundation for healthy relationships, effective communication, and a strong sense of self-worth.

Remember, every response to your baby, whether it's rocking, talking, reading, or praying, communicates love, care, and attentiveness. These simple acts of responsiveness have a profound and lasting impact on their well-being and contribute to the strong bond you share.

Let Your Baby Explore the World!

What is your baby's highest purpose? Play!

Play is one of the easiest ways to help your baby develop. Play is not just a frivolous activity; it is the primary way through which infants explore, discover, and make sense of the world around them. It is a natural and instinctive behavior that helps babies develop physically, emotionally, socially, and cognitively. During the early stages of life, babies engage in various forms of play, such as sensory play, object exploration, and social play with caregivers. Play is essential for the development of their fine and gross motor skills as they grasp, crawl, and eventually walk. These physical interactions help babies build muscle strength, coordination, and balance.

Moreover, play facilitates emotional development by allowing babies to express themselves freely. Through play, they learn to manage emotions, understand cause and effect, and build self-confidence. Simple games like peek-a-boo can teach them about trust and the concept of object permanence, contributing to their emotional security.

Social play, especially with parents or other caregivers, helps babies form secure attachments. It fosters a sense of love, trust, and connection with their primary caregivers, which is fundamental for healthy emotional and social development throughout their lives.

Cognitive development is also heavily influenced by play. Babies learn about shapes, colors, textures, and sounds through exploratory play. As they manipulate objects and observe cause-and-effect relationships, their problem-solving and critical thinking skills begin to take shape. Play serves as a foundation for future learning and helps babies become curious and engaged learners.

Play is a creative outlet for babies. It nurtures their imagination and allows them to develop symbolic thinking. Pretend play, where babies imitate everyday activities or characters, stimulates their creativity and language skills.

As babies engage in play, they also have the remarkable capacity to absorb and internalize Christian values, making play a powerful vehicle for teaching them about God's love, compassion, and grace. Parents can actively integrate Christian values into a baby's playtime. For example, they can incorporate songs and rhymes with Christian messages, read Bible stories using colorful picture books, and use toys that depict characters from biblical narratives. This reinforces the importance of faith and helps babies associate positive and joyful experiences with Christian teachings.

In today's fast-paced world, there is a growing tendency to prioritize structured learning and academic achievement from an early age.

However, play is not in conflict with learning; rather, it is the very foundation upon which learning is built. Babies learn best when they are actively engaged in the joyous exploration of their environment through play.

A baby's highest purpose is play. It is not just a pastime but a vital mechanism for growth and development. Play nurtures physical, emotional, social, and cognitive development, forming the basis for future learning and shaping a child's overall well-being. As parents, embracing and encouraging the power of play allows us to support our babies in reaching their greatest potential during these foundational years of life.

Discovering the World through the Senses

God has given our babies five wonderful senses to discover and explore His creation. Supporting your baby's sensory development helps them reach important milestones while teaching them to appreciate the beauty of God's world.

Taking your baby outside is one of the easiest ways to engage their senses. Your baby can watch clouds move across the sky, feel a gentle breeze, or follow birds as they fly. These simple moments in nature help your baby learn while experiencing God's creation.

At home, you can incorporate sensory experiences into your daily routine. During playtime, let your baby explore different materials like crinkly fabrics, soft blankets, and baby-safe textured toys. An unbreakable mirror helps them learn about facial expressions. Simple geometric shapes and bright colors, found in everyday toys and books, help develop visual skills. Most of these experiences can come from items you already have at home.

Sound is another important part of your baby's development. Classical music can be both calming and stimulating. Hymns and spiritual songs introduce them to the music of our faith. Natural sounds, from rainfall to birds singing, help them learn to listen to God's creation.

The best sensory experiences often happen naturally throughout your day. Whether you are doing laundry, making dinner, or going for a walk, there are many safe ways to help your baby explore with their senses. These simple moments support their development, your connection with them, and their growing awareness of God's presence in everyday life.

Meeting Your Baby Where They Are

In the first twelve months of life, infants undergo tremendous growth and development. However, every child is unique, and their development may not follow a rigid timeline. While some infants may achieve certain milestones at a particular age, others may take more time or reach them earlier. It's crucial for parents, caregivers, and healthcare professionals to understand and appreciate these individual variations and meet babies where they are in their developmental process.

Babies may show variations in their development due to a combination of genetic factors, environmental influences, and individual temperament. Some infants might reach physical milestones like rolling over or crawling earlier than others, while others may excel in language development or cognitive skills. These variations may be normal and shouldn't be a cause for concern unless accompanied by specific red flags or delays in multiple areas of development.

Premature babies, born before thirty-seven weeks of gestation, may require extra time to catch up with their full-term peers. Prematurity can impact various aspects of development, including motor skills, language, and cognitive abilities. Additionally, some infants may experience developmental delays or disabilities due to various medical or neurological conditions. Early intervention and support services can be instrumental in addressing these challenges and promoting optimal development.

Meeting babies where they are and using an individualized approach in their developmental process is crucial for several reasons:

- **Support and encouragement:** Recognizing and acknowledging each baby's unique progress fosters a positive and supportive environment. Encouraging their efforts, regardless of their pace, boosts their confidence and motivation to explore and learn.

- **Reducing stress and anxiety:** Comparing a baby's development to others can lead to unnecessary stress and anxiety for parents. Understanding that individual variations are normal helps parents embrace their child's journey with greater peace of mind.

- **Tailored learning and interaction:** Treating each baby as an individual allows parents to adapt their interactions and learning opportunities to suit the child's specific interests and abilities. This personalized approach can be more engaging and beneficial for the baby.

- **Early identification of concerns:** By observing and understanding a baby's unique development, parents and healthcare professionals can identify potential areas of concern or developmental delays early on. Early intervention can significantly improve outcomes and address developmental challenges effectively.

- **Appreciating diversity:** Embracing the diversity in children's development teaches us to appreciate and celebrate differences. Each child's unique journey enriches our understanding of human potential and the richness of developmental pathways.

When to Seek Professional Advice

While variations in development are normal, certain warning signs may indicate the need for professional evaluation:

- Lack of eye contact or response to sounds by six months

- Not babbling or making vocal sounds by nine months

- Unable to crawl or sit up independently by twelve months

- Does not respond to their name or show social engagement by twelve months

- Experiences significant loss of previously acquired developmental skills

As every child develops uniquely, these guidelines are meant to support, not alarm, parents in monitoring their baby's growth. However, if parents or caregivers notice any of these red flags or have concerns about their baby's development, seeking guidance from a pediatrician or early intervention specialist is essential. Timely recognition and intervention are associated with improved quality of life outcomes for the short and long term. Occupational, speech, physical, and applied behavior analysis (ABA) therapies are available with experts to guide you and your child. Such resources can contribute to a balanced plan to nurture your child's whole health with a uniquely developed plan.

Every baby's developmental journey is unique and shaped by various factors. It is vital for parents, caregivers, and healthcare professionals to meet babies where they are in their development process, recognizing and appreciating individual variations. By offering support, encouragement, and personalized interactions, we can nurture each child's potential and create an environment that celebrates the beauty of diversity in human development. Early identification of developmental concerns, when needed, allows for timely intervention and the best possible outcomes for all children. Should any developmental challenges arise, remember that our faith provides the foundation that helps us face these situations with hope, knowing that God walks this path with us.

In Summary

Supporting our children's development requires attention to their physical, cognitive, emotional, and spiritual growth. St. Gianna, who balanced her medical practice with motherhood, provides us with a beautiful example of how these aspects of health are intertwined. She recognized that a home filled with love, joy, and faith was fundamental to her children's complete development.

The spiritual dimension of parenting connects and strengthens all other aspects of development. The fruits of the Holy Spirit give us practical guidance for nurturing our children's growth. When we parent with these fruits in mind, we help our children understand they are deeply loved by their earthly parents and their heavenly Father.

Every interaction with our babies matters, from those first precious skin-to-skin cuddles to watching them explore God's creation with wonder. The way we respond to their cries, engage them in play, and expose them to new experiences shapes not just their development but their understanding of God's love. When we attend to our children's needs with consistency and care, we create an environment where they can grow in body, mind and spirit.

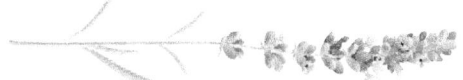

READ: *"If the Spirit of the one who raised Jesus from the dead dwells in you, the one who raised Christ from the dead will give life to your mortal bodies also, through his Spirit that dwells in you."* (Romans 8:11)

MEDITATE: What fruits of the Holy Spirit is God calling you to foster and grow?

PRAY: Breathe in me, O Holy Spirit, that my thoughts may all
be holy. Act in me, O Holy Spirit, that my work, too, may be holy.
Draw my heart, O Holy Spirit, that I love but what is holy.
Strengthen me, O Holy Spirit, to defend all that is holy.
Guard me, then, O Holy Spirit, that I always may be holy. Amen.
—Attributed to St. Augustine

LISTEN: "Spirit of the Living God" by Vertical Worship

RESOLVE: Pray for the Holy Spirit to ripen the twelve fruits in you.

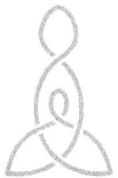

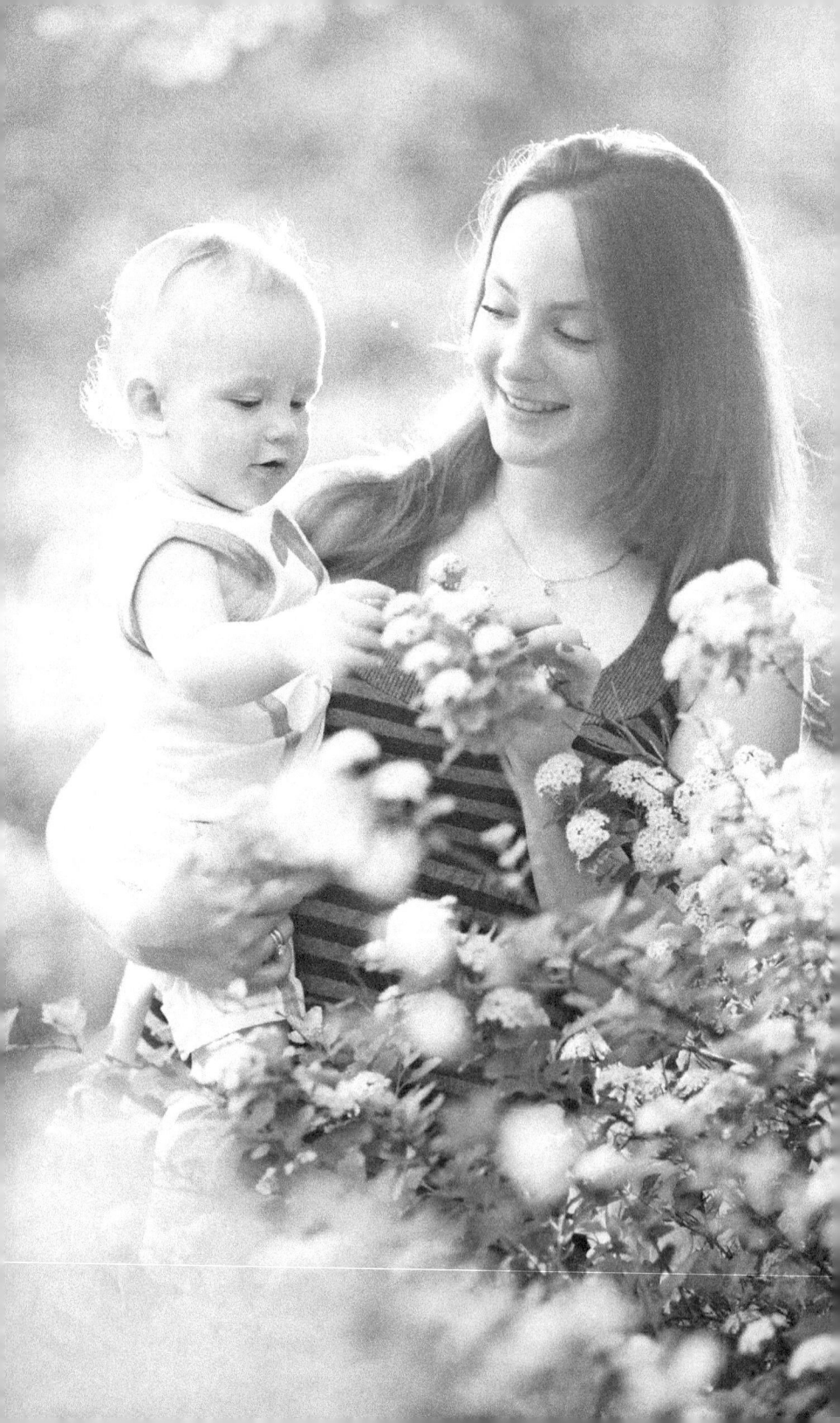

CHAPTER 14

All for His Glory

God calls each of us to embrace a life of whole health for our children and ourselves. He desires for our minds, bodies, spirits, and hearts to flourish in a way that glorifies Him and prepares us for eternity with Him. With His guidance, we can be the women He has called us to be and nourish our children and families in a way that draws us and them closer to Him.

As mothers, we often feel pulled in countless directions, and the evil one seeks to use these distractions to derail us from our purpose. Satan's attacks are particularly aimed at us because we say "yes" to new life and take on the sacred responsibility of guiding our children to love and serve Jesus. It is essential that we remain focused on our ultimate goal: bringing ourselves and our families to heaven.

Can you imagine the joy of that day when we can rejoice and dance in heaven with Jesus, Mary, and all our loved ones? This vision fills me with hope and strengthens my resolve.

The Creator of the universe knows each of us by name, calls us His beloved, and wants to foster a relationship with us. His Son, Jesus, desires to walk alongside and shepherd us so that we never feel alone.

The Holy Spirit invites us to call upon Him to guide us, reminding us of the gifts He has given us.

This journey is a lifelong quest, a continual seeking of God and aligning ourselves with His will so we may ultimately be with Him in His kingdom. The beautiful reality is that God does not want us to simply wait for heaven; He longs to be with us here and now. He desires to be invited into every aspect of our lives, offering His presence as our source of strength as we navigate the challenges of this world.

St. Martha Shows Us How

The story of St. Martha is a familiar one. It used to perplex me and make me feel uncomfortable because I am so much like St. Martha. I often wondered, "Haven't we all been called to serve?" Service is a natural inclination for me. However, my disordered need to always stay busy and fill every moment left my heart unsettled and my mind restless.

St. Martha shows us how to open our hearts to Jesus, reorder our priorities, and embrace obedience. She was once a woman "anxious and worried about many things" (Luke 10:41). Martha's actions of serving others and showing hospitality stemmed from a place of good intentions, but they distracted her from what truly matters: the presence and truth of Jesus. Her willingness to be open to Jesus' gentle rebuke reveals her willingness to reflect and reorder her priorities. A transformation began and a richer relationship with Jesus was born. She accepted His invitation to pause, listen, and draw strength from being in His presence.

Through prayer and a connection with Jesus, her faith becomes evident when she faces the death of her brother Lazarus (see John 11). When Jesus arrives, Martha goes out to meet Him immediately, while Mary stays behind. Her words to Jesus reflect both her grief and her faith: "Lord, if you had been here, my brother would not have died. [But] even now I know that whatever you ask from God, God will give you" (John 11:2–22).

In this exchange, Martha's deepening relationship with Jesus is clear. Her faith in His divine authority allows her to find strength even amid her sorrow. When Jesus declares, "I am the resurrection and the life," Martha responds with one of the most profound confessions of faith in the Gospels: "Yes, Lord. I have come to believe that you are the Messiah, the Son of God, the one who is coming into the world" (John 11:25–27). Through her relationship with Jesus, Martha receives the grace to surrender her doubts and fears, trusting in His will. Through this grace, her obedience becomes not a burden but a natural response of love and faith. Like Martha, when we nurture our relationship with Jesus, we find the strength to reorder our priorities and place our trust in Him above all else. We are called to profess this belief in word and action every day.

St. Martha teaches us that true service begins not in doing work for the sake of getting things done, but in being present and serving those God presents to us as Jesus would. We must first listen to His voice and draw on His grace. Like Martha, we are called to choose the "one thing": a life rooted in love, trust, and devotion to Christ.

> *"There is need of only one thing. Mary has chosen*
> *the better part and it will not be taken from her."*
> —Luke 10:42

Deepening Our Relationship with God through Prayer

So, how do we grow in a relationship with God? The same way we nurture relationships with our spouse, family, friends, colleagues, and fellow parishioners: by spending time together and remaining curious about one another. We slow down, open our hearts, become vulnerable, and engage in listening and responding. This divine conversation we call prayer is the foundation of our relationship with God.

For a long time, I saw prayer in a limited way, viewing it only as a means to praise, thank, ask, or seek guidance from God. I didn't see prayer as a way to simply grow my relationship with God, to find peace, rest, and nourishment. Now I understand why prayer is one of the four pillars of the Catholic Church. We must pray to learn about and grow closer to God. I used to find myself getting overwhelmed with questions: Am I doing it right? Am I grateful enough? Can God hear me? Over time, I realized the Our Father and the Rosary, prayers I had learned in childhood, were the perfect place to start. These prayers ground us and bring us back to the core of whose we are and what we believe. They give us an opportunity to come back to where God is waiting lovingly and patiently for us.

The Our Father: The Perfect Prayer

The Our Father is a prayer many of us have recited since childhood and often say without really thinking of the words. Yet it holds profound meaning. Jesus Himself taught this prayer in Matthew 6:9–15, offering us a powerful connection to God.

The opening words, "Our Father, who art in heaven," remind us of God's majesty and our ultimate call to be with Him in heaven. The *Catechism* teaches that His presence also dwells in the hearts of the just, making this phrase a proclamation of both His greatness and His closeness to us.

"Hallowed be thy name" acknowledges God's holiness and asks Him to reveal His glory. "Thy kingdom come" is a plea for His divine will to unfold on earth. As the *Catechism* states, we pray for God's reign to transform our world and our hearts and we look forward to "Christ's return and the final coming of the Reign of God" (*CCC*, 2859).

"Thy will be done on earth as it is in heaven" expresses our desire to align with God's plan. We ask for the grace to accept His truth and live according to His will.

"Give us this day our daily bread" refers to both physical and spiritual nourishment. Our true sustenance is the Word of God and the Body of Christ (see *CCC*, 2861). Even if we cannot attend Mass, Scripture is always available to feed our souls, just as God provided manna for the Israelites in the desert.

"Forgive us our trespasses as we forgive those who trespass against us" asks for God's mercy while reminding us to show mercy to others. This reflects Matthew 5:7: "Blessed are the merciful, for they shall receive mercy."

"Lead us not into temptation" can be misunderstood, as God does not lead us into sin. Instead, we seek His strength to resist trials and avoid the snares of the enemy.

"Deliver us from evil" is a plea for God's protection against sin and all that separates us from Him.

The Our Father is more than words; it is a blueprint for faith, trust, and surrender to God's will. Through this prayer, we acknowledge His holiness, seek His guidance, and express our dependence on Him.

The Beauty of the Rosary

As a child, the Rosary felt like an obligation to me. In college, I rediscovered its comfort, often whispering Hail Marys as I drifted off to sleep. Years later, I came to understand its richness: the mysteries, the embedded Scripture, and the unfolding story of Christ's life.

Meditating on the sacred mysteries while praying the Rosary brings peace and clarity of purpose in life. One particular mystery, the Fourth Joyful Mystery of the Presentation in the Temple, has profoundly touched my heart. Mary and Joseph, though without need for purification or redemption, humbly followed Jewish law. Simeon and Anna, recognizing the infant Jesus, rejoiced in God's fulfilled promise. Even as a baby, Jesus was already offering Himself to the world.

Praying the Rosary gets me through performing the chores I would rather not have to do such as laundry or driving in traffic. It keeps me focused on connecting with Jesus' mother and praying for her intercession.

Expanding Your Spiritual Life

As we walk our unique spiritual paths, God gently reveals new ways for us to pray. He knows our hearts and meets us where we are, preparing us for growth in seasons we never could have planned for ourselves. Over time, I have discovered different rhythms of prayer that help me stay rooted and open to His grace. Mornings often begin with the daily reading from the Laudate app while I stretch or do simple floor exercises, offering my body and my day to the Lord. During commutes, I pray the Rosary along with Jonathan Roumie on the Hallow app. It helps center my mind in peace. On my lunch break, I'll often turn to the Divine Mercy Chaplet or the Litany of Trust, short but powerful ways to pause and reconnect with God's mercy. In the evenings, I open Scripture and journal a short prayer of gratitude, my petitions, and a request for guidance. Beyond these daily practices, I try to carve out intentional time each week for deeper forms of prayer like lectio divina, visio divina, or reflecting on music paired with Scripture. I'm also deeply nourished by my monthly women's prayer group and reading the writings of the saints, especially those who have walked the path of ordinary holiness. Through these rhythms, I've come to realize that prayer isn't about performance; it's about presence. Like St. Martha, who learned to realign her busy heart with God's will, I too am learning to sit at His feet, day by day.

KATHRYN—PRAYER PRACTICES

Like many Catholics, my early prayer life centered around the beautiful traditional prayers I learned in childhood. Though I said some unscripted prayers to God such as thanking him for blessings in my life or asking for intercessions for the needs of myself or others, most of my prayers were rote prayers I learned in childhood.

As my faith has matured, I have been able to explore other types of prayer and have become more comfortable just spending time with God. As I've entered different seasons in my life, my prayer practices have changed and evolved. The Holy Spirit often guides me to different forms of prayer depending on what my heart needs in a particular moment. Though I use many types of prayers regularly, three prayer practices are my favorites: Eucharistic adoration, lectio divina, and guided prayer.

One of God's greatest gifts to our parish is a twenty-four-hour perpetual adoration chapel. One of my favorite ways to pray is to go to adoration and just be with Jesus in the Eucharist. Though I have several different guides and prayer resources for adoration, often I just like to sit in silence and let peace wash over me. There have been occasions when I am out doing errands or dropping one of my children off at school (which happens to be across the street from the chapel!) and I'll feel called to go to adoration for a few minutes. I almost always leave feeling calmer and restored.

Lectio divina is another prayer practice I enjoy. Reading a short passage and meditating on that reading can be very profound. It helps me realize that Scripture truly is alive and meaningful to every part of my life. Now that our children are older, my husband and I have started to do a modified version of *lectio divina* at home in the evenings with them. We pick a passage and read it slowly three times. We focus on words that are relevant to us, phrases that are significant, and then discuss what the passage means to us and how we can apply it to our lives. I love hearing our children's perspectives on each verse or passage.

A third type of prayer that I use daily is guided prayer, often with the Hallow app. This type of prayer offers insights I may not have thought of on my own. Podcasts such as *Bible in a Year* by Father Mike Schmitz have encouraged and challenged me to delve into Scripture in new ways. These guided formats offer time for prayer as well as education, which has benefited me immensely.

Remember that prayer does not always require perfect circumstances or long, uninterrupted periods of time. Feeding your baby or watching them sleep can be a time of thanksgiving. Prayer does not have to be long to glorify God and to grow in your relationship with Him. Though your days may seem hectic, finding those little moments to pray can help you find peace.

The Power of the Sacraments and the Call to Sacramental Living

The sacraments are more than rituals; they are encounters with the living God. Without a relationship with Christ, they risk becoming routine rather than transformative. My journey back to a deeper faith began with recognizing the sacraments as lifelines to God's grace. The sacraments are the path to reconnecting with God and the way for nourishing our whole health.

Each Baptism in our family has been a deeply sacred moment. When Evan and Charlie were baptized, I was overwhelmed knowing original sin was washed away and Christ's light was ignited in their hearts. Baptism is more than a rite of passage; it is a transformation of the soul.

In Baptism we give our children back to God and declare that our child belongs to him. We invite the Holy Spirit to dwell within them, guide them, and strengthen them. Baptism welcomes them into the Body of Christ, uniting them with the Church. As St. Paul tells us in 1 Corinthians 12:12–13:

> "As a body is one though it has many parts, and all the parts of the body, though many, are one body, so also Christ. For in one Spirit we were all baptized into one body, whether Jews or Greeks, slaves or free persons, and we were all given to drink of one Spirit."

I will never forget the day of Evan's baptism. While holding my sweet baby, feeling his soft head against my cheek, and seeing the sunlight stream through the stained glass windows, I knew at that moment that the Spirit of the Lord was upon him. A choice had been made; he was God's child. And when it came time for Charles to be baptized, Keith and I took the preparation classes together. I held Charlie in the back of the room, listening to the beautiful truths of our faith.

Sisters in Christ, I urge you to baptize your children. Let the waters of life wash over them, making them part of the Body of Christ.

Show your faithful obedience, just as Mary and Joseph did. Give your most precious loves back to God, recognizing that they have always belonged to Him. And take heart, knowing that the God who created them rejoices as they are brought into His family, loved beyond measure for all eternity.

On the day of Charlie's baptism, the Holy Spirit deepened my husband's and my desire to seek the Lord and live fully in His grace. We knew we had to continue to truly practice our Catholic faith and receive God's grace through the sacraments if we wanted our family to live the Christian life. Each sacrament we receive strengthens our bond to Christ, like branches firmly connected to the true vine. In the sacraments, we experience the ongoing flow of God's grace, and we are able to grow in faith, courage, and love. He then calls us to shine and pour out to others what he has given by living a sacramental life.

Living a sacramental life means continually receiving God's grace through the sacraments, which strengthen and nourish us for the journey. The Eucharist feeds our souls with His very presence, and through Confession, He restores us to His love. The sacraments equip us to be His witnesses, to bring His love to those who need it most, and to reflect His invisible grace through our visible lives.

The grace we receive through the sacraments strengthens us for the beautiful but sometimes challenging journey of raising our children in the faith. I learned this firsthand when bringing my own infant to Mass. When Charlie was less than three months old, we felt like we had hit the jackpot with taking him to church. He seemed to love the music and would quickly fall asleep and stay quiet throughout the Mass. At about four months of age, he suddenly decided Mass was not a time to be quiet. He started crying so much that we moved from the main sanctuary to the cry room—and then out the back doors! He quickly calmed down once we were outside, and we decided he was probably worn out enough to go to lunch. As soon as we ordered our food, the crying started up again. A kind couple who had seen us at Mass offered words that still encourage me today: "We saw you at church, and we see you here. Don't give up. Keep going out, but most especially, keep going to Mass."

Their kind encouragement reminded me that our *perseverance in faith matters*, not just for ourselves but for our children. The Lord lifts us up through the sacraments, His presence, and His people, even during those challenging moments. So take heart, dear mothers, and bring your little ones to Mass. Your presence there, even on difficult days, is a beautiful witness.

Living a sacramental life means trusting that Jesus will meet us on our journey when we seek to do His will. He calls us to approach Him, humble ourselves before Him, and kneel at His feet in reverence and love. He desires our praise, our homage, and our trust. Through His power, we find the courage to show His love to the world.

Called to Help Carry One Another's Crosses

As Jesus made His way to Calvary, Simon of Cyrene was pressed into service to help carry the cross (see Mark 15:21). Through this unexpected encounter, Simon became part of salvation history, witnessing Christ's sacrifice directly and sharing in His burden.

Like Simon, we are called to help carry the crosses of fellow mothers on their journey. Sometimes this means offering encouragement to the mom with the crying baby at Mass, sharing our own struggles and victories in faith, or simply being present when another mother needs support. These seemingly small acts of service become powerful testimonies of Christ's love.

Jesus tells us, "Do not be afraid," and calls us to share His love with the world. When we reach out to support another mother, share our own faith journey, or witness to His grace in our lives, we become His hands and feet in the world. By staying connected to Him through prayer and the sacraments, we find the courage to reach out and help others find their way to Him.

Let us not be afraid to go forth and live a sacramental life, connected to the true vine, bearing fruit through His grace, and showing the world the love and mercy of Christ. With prayer as our foundation and the sacraments as our nourishment, we are called to witness to others and bring them to Him.

In Summary

Sisters in Christ, everything we do as mothers can be offered up for God's glory. From early morning feedings to bedtime prayers, each moment is a chance to draw closer to Him and lead our children toward heaven. Like St. Martha, when we reorder our priorities and place Christ at the center, our lives reflect His glory.

Through prayer, we open our hearts to His presence. Through the sacraments, we receive grace to see His presence in every moment of our day. When we embrace sacramental living, our homes become places where His light shines and our children witness what it means to live for God's glory.

May we continue to encourage one another on this journey, remembering that our ultimate purpose is to glorify God in all we do. In giving Him glory through a life rooted in prayer and the sacraments, we help our children discover their purpose: to know, love, and serve Him in this world and be prepared for a life with Him forever in heaven.

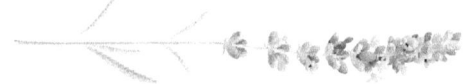

READ: *"Train the young in the way they should go; even when old, they will not swerve from it."* (Proverbs 22:6)

MEDITATE: Imagine yourself standing before Jesus and hear Him say to you, "Well done, My beloved daughter—welcome home."

PRAY: Lord God, from You every family in Heaven and on earth takes its name. Father, You are love and life. Through Your Son, Jesus Christ, born of woman, and through the Holy Spirit, the fountain of divine charity, grant that every family on earth may become for each successive generation a true shrine of life and love.
   – Grant that Your grace may guide the thoughts and actions of husbands and wives for the good of their families and of all the families in the world.
   – Grant that the young may find in the family solid support for their human dignity and for their growth in truth and love.
   – Grant that love, strengthened by the grace of the sacrament of marriage, may prove mightier than all the weaknesses and trials through which our families sometimes pass.
   – Through the intercession of the Holy Family of Nazareth, grant that the Church may fruitfully carry out her worldwide mission in the family and through the family. We ask this of You, Who is life, truth and love with the Son and the Holy Spirit. Amen.
— Prayer for Families, St. John Paul II[57]

LISTEN: "Set a Fire" by Jesus Culture

RESOLVE: Sing "This Little Light of Mine" to your baby and really focus on the lyrics and their challenge to us.

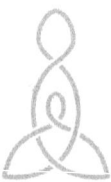

---

57   *Prayer of St. John Paul II for All Families*, Aleteia.org, https://aleteia.org/2017/12/31/prayer-of-st-john-paul-ii-for-all-families.

Conclusion

Throughout this book, we have explored the fundamental principles of nurturing babies, integrating essential child-care practices with faith formation. We have discovered how to create an environment that fosters growth and development: by prioritizing what truly matters, adapting with grace to changing circumstances, and expressing love consistently.

As a new parent, it is easy to be overwhelmed by the plethora of information and advice available. In this book, we have stressed the significance of returning to the basics of child care. Your baby's health and well-being flourish when built on simple but essential foundations: a safe and loving environment, proper nourishment, adequate sleep, and good hygiene. As you embark on this journey, remember that mastering the basics is not about perfection, but rather about consistently providing the love and care your baby needs to thrive.

We have explored the often-neglected topic of faith formation for you and your children. Cultivating your baby's spiritual development can have a profound impact on their overall well-rounded growth. Providing a sense of spiritual connection instills values, compassion, and a sense of purpose in your little one's life. Incorporating faith-based practices, rituals, or teachings into your daily routine lays the groundwork for a strong moral compass and emotional resilience as they grow.

Parenthood is not a one-size-fits-all journey. Each baby is unique, and so are their needs. By prioritizing what is most important for both you and your baby, you can create a personalized approach to child care that aligns with your family's values, lifestyle, and circumstances. Embrace flexibility and be willing to adapt as your baby grows and their needs change. Trust your instincts and let them guide you in making the best decisions for your child.

Implementing, assessing, and adjusting are integral parts of the parenting process. As you put the principles and ideas from this book into practice, be open to assessing their effectiveness. Observe how your baby responds and evaluate whether adjustments are needed. Remember, parenting is a continuous learning experience, and being attuned to your baby's cues will guide you in providing the care and support they require.

Throughout this journey, grant yourself the space and grace to grow as a parent. It is normal to face challenges, make mistakes, and experience moments of doubt. Be compassionate with yourself, knowing that you are doing the best you can with the love you have for your child. Seek support from friends, family, or parenting communities when needed, and remember that you are not alone on this path.

Never underestimate the power of love in your baby's life! Express your affection openly and frequently, saying those three simple yet profound words, "I love you," to your little one. Love is the cornerstone of a baby's well-being, providing them with a strong emotional foundation that will shape their future relationships and overall happiness.

Nurturing your baby's whole health is a multifaceted journey that requires dedication, love, and understanding. By focusing on the basics of child care, tending to their spiritual development, prioritizing what matters most, and being flexible in your approach, you will create an environment in which your baby can thrive. Implementing, assessing, and adjusting with space and grace will allow you to continuously refine your parenting skills and adapt to your baby's changing needs.

As Scripture reminds us, "I can do all things in him who strengthens me" (Philippians 4:13, RSVCE). This promise extends to your vocation as a mother. Through it all, let God be your guiding light, for in Him, you will find the strength and joy to embrace every moment of this beautiful journey called parenthood. In nurturing your child's relationship with God, you are fulfilling one of your most sacred duties as a Catholic parent: helping your baby grow not just in body and mind, but in spirit, drawing ever closer to our loving Father.

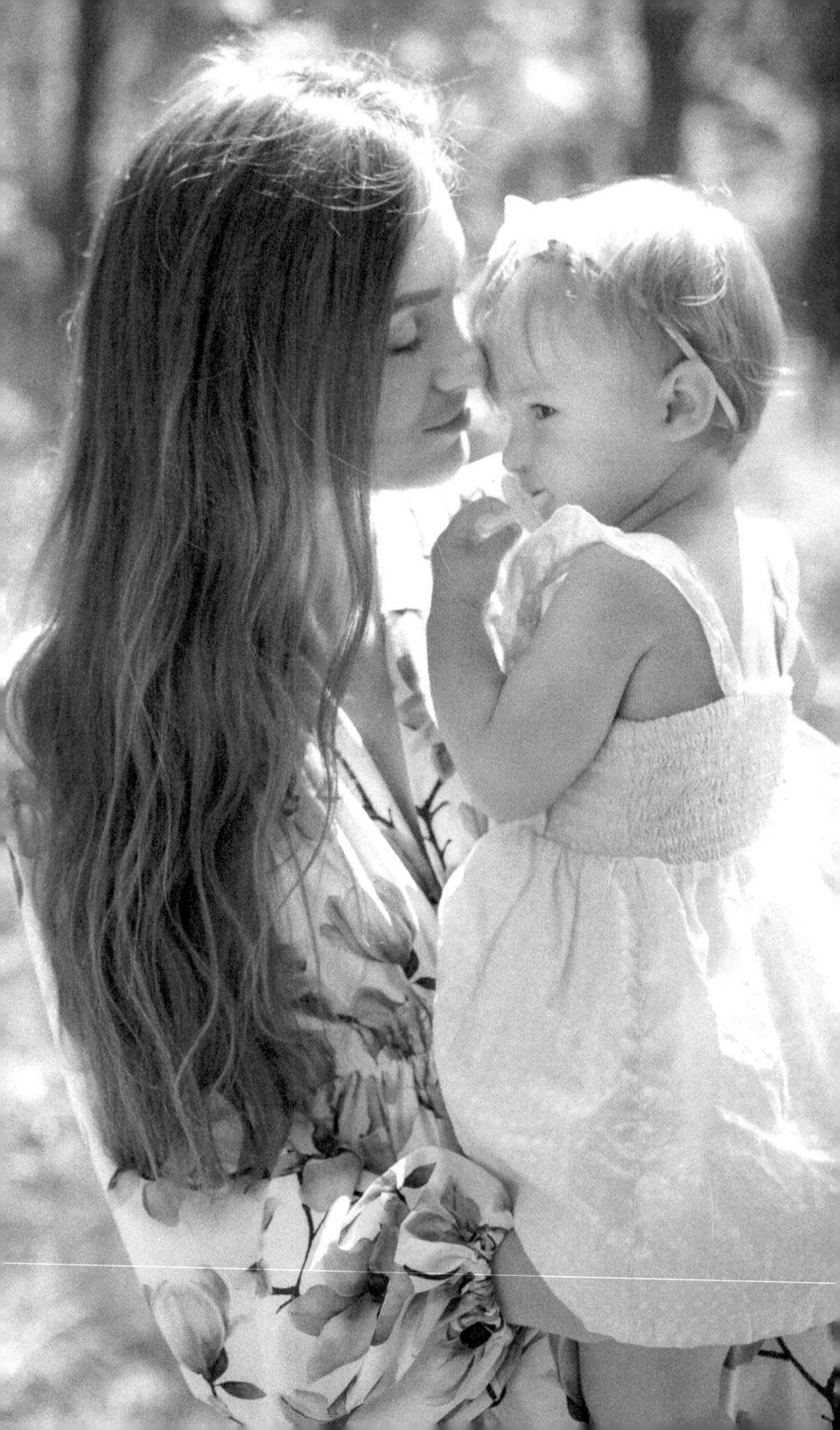

Appendices

Appendix I:
Choosing a Pediatric Provider

Discerning a healthcare provider for your infant can be a challenging process. You want a provider who practices evidence-based medicine while also being supportive and respectful of your family's background and choices. A good pediatrician or pediatric nurse practitioner should make you feel comfortable asking questions and be someone you trust to guide your family's health decisions. The right provider should not only educate you about the latest medical evidence but also take time to listen to your concerns and explain their recommendations.

Many pediatric offices have opportunities for you to meet one or more of their providers and ask questions prior to giving birth. Some offices will hold group "meet the doctor" sessions where you can come learn about the practice and meet some (or all) of the providers. Other offices may offer prenatal appointments where you can meet a provider individually. Either of these options are great to consider as you are exploring your choices.

During your search, consider asking about their stance on key issues that matter to you, such as their approach to vaccination, antibiotic use, and preventive care. It is perfectly acceptable to ask potential pediatricians about their medical philosophy during a meet-and-greet session or prenatal visit—after all, this person will be a crucial partner in your child's healthcare journey. Don't be afraid to keep searching until you find a pediatric provider whose medical philosophy and approach align with your own values and parenting style.

The following questions and tips are practical things to consider when choosing a pediatric provider for your family:

- **How far away is the office from your home?** You will be seeing your medical provider many times in the first year! There are typically at least seven preventative care visits in the first year of life. Additionally, there may be added visits for weight checks, feeding concerns, or sick appointments. Though there may be a wonderful provider across town, it's important to discern whether this is worth a significantly longer drive multiple times a year.

- **Will you see the same provider for each preventative care visit?** A good pediatrician, pediatric nurse practitioner, or family practice physician will get to know you and your baby over the first few visits. They will learn how your baby is growing and developing and establish a relationship with your family. If possible, it's important to see the same provider for those preventative care visits so you can build rapport. While you may need to see other providers for more urgent or same-day appointments, it's preferable to have one provider follow your baby's growth and development. This sets them up to be better able to educate you and to identify concerns.

- **What are their office hours?** Many pediatric offices now offer some evening and weekend hours. It's helpful to know whether your pediatric office offers appointments at times more convenient to working parents.

- **How does the office schedule sick appointments or same-day visits?** The first time your baby is sick can be very stressful. If you have concerns about your infant and want to see your provider, you want to be seen in a timely manner. Some pediatric offices have walk-in hours for urgent or same day visits. Other offices will have multiple reserved appointment slots for same day needs. Make sure you are aware of your office's scheduling policies. If you are scheduling an appointment, tell the scheduler all of your concerns. As a pediatrician, I always wanted to make sure I had enough time to address all issues. If there are concerns about development or chronic symptoms, it's best to be up front with the office when scheduling. Know that, sometimes, more chronic issues may need to be addressed at multiple visits or at a visit scheduled several days in advance to allow enough time.

- **How does the office handle after-hours needs?** Questions or problems inevitably seem to arise in the middle of the night or on the weekends! Find out ahead of time what your prospective pediatric office does when concerns come up after hours. Some offices provide a nurse triage line for advice when the office is closed. Other offices may have an answering service that will directly page a provider on call. Many offices may offer a hybrid system combining both nurse triage and a physician on call. Additionally, be aware that sometimes there are multiple offices sharing the same on-call service. Sometimes answering services or nurse triage programs are provided by larger systems, and these may not have direct access to your patient records. Make sure you feel comfortable with whatever your office offers.

- **What happens if your child needs to go to the emergency room or hospital?** In many areas of the country, pediatric providers no longer see their patients in the emergency room or hospital. The trend has been for hospitals to employ physicians known as hospitalists (physicians that dedicate their practice to the care of in-hospital patients). While some providers may still see their own patients in the emergency room or hospital, most pediatric providers will either practice in an office or solely in the hospital. If your child needs an emergency room or hospital, it's helpful to at least know what your pediatric provider recommends and what their individual practice policies are.

Though there are many other questions you may come up with, the suggestions above are a good starting point as you discern the best healthcare provider for your child. Most importantly, pick someone you are comfortable with and trust to guide you and your family.

Pediatricians and pediatric nurse practitioners love kids! We want to watch your child grow and are eager to help you along the journey. We want your children to succeed! Yet we all have different personalities, and we may have slightly different opinions on certain topics. If you find that you are uncomfortable with your chosen pediatric provider, don't be afraid to seek out someone new. Pray about it, ask the Holy Spirit to guide your decision, and do what is best for your family.

Appendix 2:
Intimacy after Delivery

Intimacy after childbirth is tender, complicated, and different for every mother. Let's be honest, intimacy isn't something you often hear Catholics openly talking about, especially in the messy, real-life moments of early motherhood. But it's important to talk about it. God created our bodies for love and connection. God designed marriage to reflect the union between Christ and the Church, and intimacy is a sacred part of that union. This gift is not only for creating life but also serves as a sign of love, trust, and self-giving. It is holy, and when approached with gentleness and grace, it can be healing too.

No one prepares you for how much your heart and body will change after becoming a mother. The process of returning to intimacy after birth can feel awkward. You've just walked through a life-changing and sacred experience by bringing life into the world. Creating your new normal requires love and patience.

After my boys were born, I remember feeling like my whole self belonged to others; between caring for my baby and family, there seemed to be endless demands on my time and body. My body no longer felt like my own. I loved my child deeply, and I realized I was adapting to a new self. Looking back, I was grateful when my doctor recommended waiting to resume sex. For both vaginal and C-section deliveries, most doctors recommend a four- to six-week recovery period before having intercourse again. It's important to be cleared by your medical provider before resuming sexual activity. While this waiting period is medically necessary for healing and preventing infection, it also gives moms time to prepare emotionally. Sometimes this takes months, not weeks.

After a vaginal birth, it is common to experience vaginal dryness. This is particularly true if you are breastfeeding, since lower estrogen levels contribute to dryness. Using a water-based lubricant can help reduce discomfort. It's a simple, empowering tool—not a sign that anything is wrong.

If you've had a C-section, the incision site may still be tender, and your core might feel weak. Side-lying positions or being on top can give you more control and comfort.

One thing I was not prepared for was breast tenderness. Whether from engorgement, let-down reflex, or sore nipples, my chest felt off-limits, and that's okay. It's perfectly fine to wear a bra during intimacy. Choose a soft nursing bra or something that makes you feel supported. There's no rule that says you have to bare everything to feel close.

What mattered most in our journey back to intimacy wasn't the specifics of what we did but rather the intention and patience. It became an opportunity to practice gentleness and mutual understanding. Communication, even when it felt awkward, helped us grow closer.

As you navigate this journey, remember that fertility often returns before you might expect, even while breastfeeding. Natural Family Planning (NFP) offers a beautiful way to understand your body's cycle while honoring God's design for marriage. Many Catholic couples find that NFP deepens their relationship as they practice responsible parenthood together. Your diocese or parish can connect you with local NFP instructors and support groups to guide you.[58]

Above all, remember: You are not broken. You are healing. You are allowed to take your time. Real intimacy after childbirth is not about resuming what was; it's about honoring who you are now and learning how to love in this new, beautiful season.

---

58   "Natural Family Planning," *USCCB*, https://www.usccb.org/topics/natural-family-planning.

Appendix 3:
Choosing the Right Child Care

Below are some considerations when discerning child care options for your family:

- **Start early:** Begin your search for child care options well in advance. Waiting until the last minute can add unnecessary stress. Starting early allows you to research thoroughly and visit multiple facilities to find the best fit.

- **Define your needs:** Consider your family's unique needs and preferences. Are you looking for full-time care, part-time care, or occasional babysitting? Identify essential factors like location, operating hours, and age-appropriate programs.

- **Research and gather information:** Use various resources to gather information about local child care options. Ask for recommendations from friends, family, or neighbors, and read online reviews to gain insights from other parents' experiences.

- **Visit and observe:** Schedule visits to potential child care centers or meet with individual caregivers. Observe the environment, cleanliness, and safety measures. Pay attention to the interactions between caregivers and children to gauge the level of warmth and attentiveness.

- **Ask questions:** Prepare a list of questions to ask during your visits. Inquire about the caregiver-to-child ratio, staff qualifications, safety protocols, daily routines, and how they handle emergencies. An open and transparent dialogue is crucial.

- **Check licensing and accreditation:** Ensure the child care provider is licensed and adheres to local regulations. Accredited facilities often meet higher standards of care and safety.

- **Consider the curriculum:** If the child care facility offers a structured curriculum, review it to ensure it aligns with your child's developmental needs. Look for programs that encourage learning, creativity, and social interaction.

- **Assess communication:** Determine how the child care provider communicates with parents. Regular updates and open communication are vital for staying informed about your child's progress and well-being.

- **Trust your instincts:** Pay attention to your gut feeling about a particular child care option. If something feels off or you have reservations, trust your instincts and continue exploring other options.

- **Require references:** Ask for references from other parents whose children have attended the child care center. Speaking with current or previous clients can offer valuable feedback and help you make an informed decision.

- **Set a trial period:** Consider arranging a trial period for your child to assess how they adapt to the new environment. A trial allows you to observe how your child interacts with caregivers and other children before making a long-term commitment.

- **Review policies and contracts:** Carefully review the facility's policies, including sick leave, vacation days, payment schedules, and termination clauses. Ensure you understand the terms and conditions before signing any contracts.

Remember that choosing the right child care is a significant step in your child's early development. Take the time to explore your options thoroughly and prioritize your child's safety, well-being, and overall happiness. Trust your judgment and seek child care that aligns with your family's values and needs, providing a nurturing environment for your child to thrive.

Appendix 4:
Developmental Milestones

The first year of life is filled with wonderful developmental changes for your baby. This is a period of rapid growth and progression. Below are some milestones pediatricians and developmental specialists may watch for. Keep in mind that babies progress at their own rates and the failure to meet one of these milestones does not automatically indicate cause for concern.

YOUR BABY AT TWO MONTHS

The first two months bring wonderful changes as your little one becomes more alert and responsive. Here's what you might notice:

Moving and Growing

- Your baby is gaining weight and growing longer (your pediatrician will track these changes).
- They may begin to have a bit of head control.
- During tummy time, they might start pushing up a bit.
- Those early jerky movements become smoother.

Connecting with the World

- Your baby will begin showing their first social smiles.
- Your baby will focus more on faces.
- Cooing and gurgling sounds begin to emerge.
- Your baby will begin to calm down when spoken to or picked up.
- They will start recognizing familiar voices and faces.

Learning and Thinking

- Your baby will be more alert to their surroundings.
- Your baby will watch you move around the room and track objects in a purposeful way.
- New sounds and sights catch their attention more easily.

YOUR BABY AT FOUR MONTHS

At four months, your baby's personality becomes more evident as they begin to explore their world. Here's what you might see:

Moving and Growing

- Many babies have doubled their birth weight by this age!
- Head and neck control is getting much stronger.
- Some babies begin rolling.
- They are reaching out and batting at toys and objects.

Connecting with the World

- Smiles develop into laughter and giggles.
- Your baby enjoys social interaction with familiar people.
- They can focus better now, especially on objects six to eighteen inches away.
- Colors are becoming more vivid in their world.

Learning and Thinking

- They might try to make sound in response to you speaking with them.
- Oral exploration of objects becomes common.
- Your baby starts to recognize daily routines.

YOUR BABY AT SIX MONTHS

At six months, your baby continues to develop new skills and abilities. Here is what typically happens at this age:

Moving and Growing

- Many babies now roll in both directions.
- Sitting on their own is beginning, though some support may still be needed.
- When you hold them up, they will want to "stand" on their legs.
- Your baby will grasp objects within reach, from toys to hair.

Connecting with the World

- Your baby is becoming more social, though they may prefer familiar faces.
- Some babies start getting a bit shy around unfamiliar faces.
- They may begin to enjoy playing peek-a-boo or other games.
- Their babbling includes more varied sounds and squeals.

Learning and Thinking

- They respond when you call their name.
- Objects get passed from hand to hand, often followed by oral exploration.
- Their natural curiosity leads them to explore their environment.
- Hand-eye coordination is improving daily.

YOUR BABY AT NINE MONTHS

Movement and mobility increase significantly at this age. At nine months, your baby's world is expanding rapidly as new abilities make exploration possible. Here's what you might notice:

Moving and Growing

- Many babies are crawling, though some may find different ways to move and some may skip crawling altogether.
- Sitting solo is often mastered by now.
- The pincer grasp begins to develop.

Connecting with the World

- Your baby might want to stay close to familiar caregivers.
- Stranger anxiety may increase; this is a normal developmental stage.
- Interactive games become increasingly engaging.
- Understanding of words and simple phrases increases.

Learning and Thinking

- Problem-solving skills are emerging.
- They are learning that things exist even when hidden.
- They experiment with cause and effect.
- Babbling might sound more like real conversation.

YOUR BABY AT TWELVE MONTHS

Happy first birthday! At twelve months, your baby transitions from infant to toddler—a significant developmental milestone. Here's what you might see:

Moving and Growing

- First steps may begin around this time.
- Fingers are becoming more skilled at handling small objects.
- Growth rate might slow down a bit; this is normal.
- They are getting better at judging distances.

Connecting with the World

- "Mama" and "Dada" are probably favorite words.
- They may understand simple commands such as "no" or "come here."
- Your baby may mimic your gestures and expressions.
- They begin waving and pointing to communicate.

Learning and Thinking

- Games like hide-and-seek with toys become engaging.
- They understand simple cause and effect.
- Active exploration of their environment becomes a primary focus.
- They learn from watching everything you do.

Remember, every baby develops at their own pace. These milestones are general guidelines, not strict rules. If you have concerns about your baby's development, your pediatrician is always there to help.

Resources: https://www.cdc.gov/ncbddd/actearly/milestones/index.html
https://www.cdc.gov/ncbddd/actearly/milestones-app.html
https://pathways.org/track/milestones

Appendix 5:
Chocolate Depression Cake

This recipe gets its name because this type of cake was popular during the Great Depression when families didn't have the resources to use butter or eggs. It works wonderfully as a sheet cake, cupcakes, or even layer cakes. Most commonly, I have made one batch to make three short eight-inch round cakes that I make into a layer cake. They are slightly more fragile and light than a typical bakery layer cake, so be careful when stacking!

Ingredients:

- 3 cups flour
- 2 cups sugar
- scant 1 teaspoon salt
- 2 teaspoons baking soda
- 10 level tablespoons unsweetened cocoa (not Dutch processed)

- 2 teaspoons vanilla
- 3/4 cup vegetable oil
- 2 tablespoons white vinegar
- 2 cups cold water

Preparation:

Sift dry ingredients into a large mixing bowl. Mix wet ingredients together. Add wet ingredients to dry and mix with a large spoon until smooth. Spoon into a greased and floured 13x9x2-inch baking pan. Bake at 350° for 30 to 40 minutes until a pick inserted in the center comes out clean (or almost clean). Frost with your favorite frosting.

If you make cupcakes, the baking time will be only fifteen to twenty minutes. Watch carefully so they do not overcook. Round eight-inch cake pans also will take less time than a sheet pan—usually about twenty minutes—so watch carefully.

About the Authors

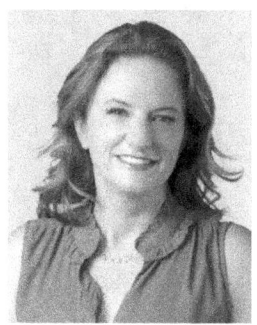

Nicole Lea

Nicole Lea, RN, MSN, CPNP, CPHQ, completed her bachelor of science in Nursing at Emory University. In 2005, after practicing as a bedside nurse in the emergency department and pediatric cardiology intensive and acute care units, she became a Certified Pediatric Nurse Practitioner. For sixteen years she cared for children with complex medical needs, including stem cell transplant and lung transplant recipients. She currently works on projects that promote healthcare quality and patient safety.

Nicole lives with her husband, two children, and two pups in Houston, Texas. She enjoys being with family, gardening, or traveling to explore God's glorious outdoors. Nicole and her family are active in their local parish and she co-leads a women's prayer group. By God's divine grace, Nicole met Kathryn at a *Walking with Purpose* conference at exactly the right time! She is passionate about inspiring women to follow God's heart and live with boldness and hope.

Invite Nicole to speak to your women's or moms' group about how to *Nurture Whole Health* for themselves and their children. Free faith-rooted, evidence-informed content and resources for caring for babies, children, and teenagers are available at **HelloEema.com**. Contact Nicole at **nicole@helloeema.com**.

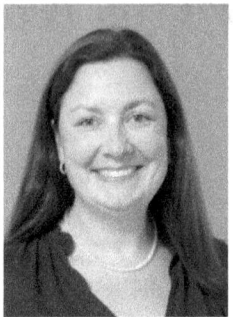

Kathryn Italia

Kathryn Italia, MD, completed her medical education at Thomas Jefferson University in Philadelphia and pediatric residency at duPont Hospital for Children (now Nemours Children's Hospital Wilmington). She practiced pediatrics for fourteen years, caring for hundreds of families before transitioning to focus on her own family in 2022. Her experience in primary care brought an essential perspective to this book about nurturing children's whole health.

Kathryn lives with her husband and three children in Pennsylvania, where they share a love for travel and outdoor adventures, especially in the mountains where God's majesty is on display. She is active in her parish community and women's Bible study groups. At a national Catholic women's conference, she met Nicole, and their shared vision of faith-centered motherhood led to this collaboration. She considers herself blessed to combine her medical background with her faith to help other mothers on their parenting journey.

Continuing the Journey

As you reach the final pages of this book, we want to take a moment to honor your journey on this sacred, beautiful, and often challenging path of motherhood. You're not just raising a child; you're nurturing a whole person in body, mind, heart and soul. Through this calling, God also wants to continue to nurture and transform you too.

Throughout this book, we've explored how to care for your child's physical, emotional, cognitive, and spiritual development, while also tending to your own well-being. These aspects of health are not separate but beautifully intertwined, and your intentional care in each one creates an environment where love, faith, and growth can flourish. This often unseen daily work is where authentic holiness takes root.

But this journey doesn't end here. God is still calling us into deeper relationship with Him, inviting us to pray without ceasing, and to allow our lives to become a witness of His love, just as Mary and the saints show us.

If you're looking for ongoing support, we invite you to join us at *Hello Eema*, a space created to walk alongside mothers like you. The name "Eema" represents "mama" and is what Jesus calls Mary in The Chosen. It's a tender reminder that we're all beloved daughters of God following in our heavenly Mother's footsteps. "Hello" is our greeting of recognition and hope: You are seen and not alone.

At *Hello Eema*, you'll discover practical guidance grounded in faith, enriched by expertise in nursing and medical sciences, and shaped by real motherhood experiences. We offer resources to help you navigate your child's physical, emotional, cognitive, and spiritual development while nurturing a growing, heartfelt relationship with Christ.

This space isn't about achieving perfect motherhood; it's about allowing God to continually shape your heart and your home. He gently chisels away fear, fatigue, and doubt, and replaces them with courage, peace, and purpose.

Remember, we were never meant to walk this path alone. The Holy Spirit, our Blessed Mother, the saints in Heaven, and us, your sisters in Christ, are with you every step of the way.

THANK YOU

for letting us walk with you in these pages. We pray you'll continue the journey with us at **www.helloeema.com**, where we grow stronger together in faith, supporting each other toward our shared destination: eternal life with Christ.

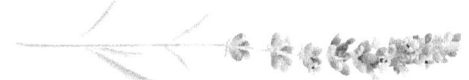

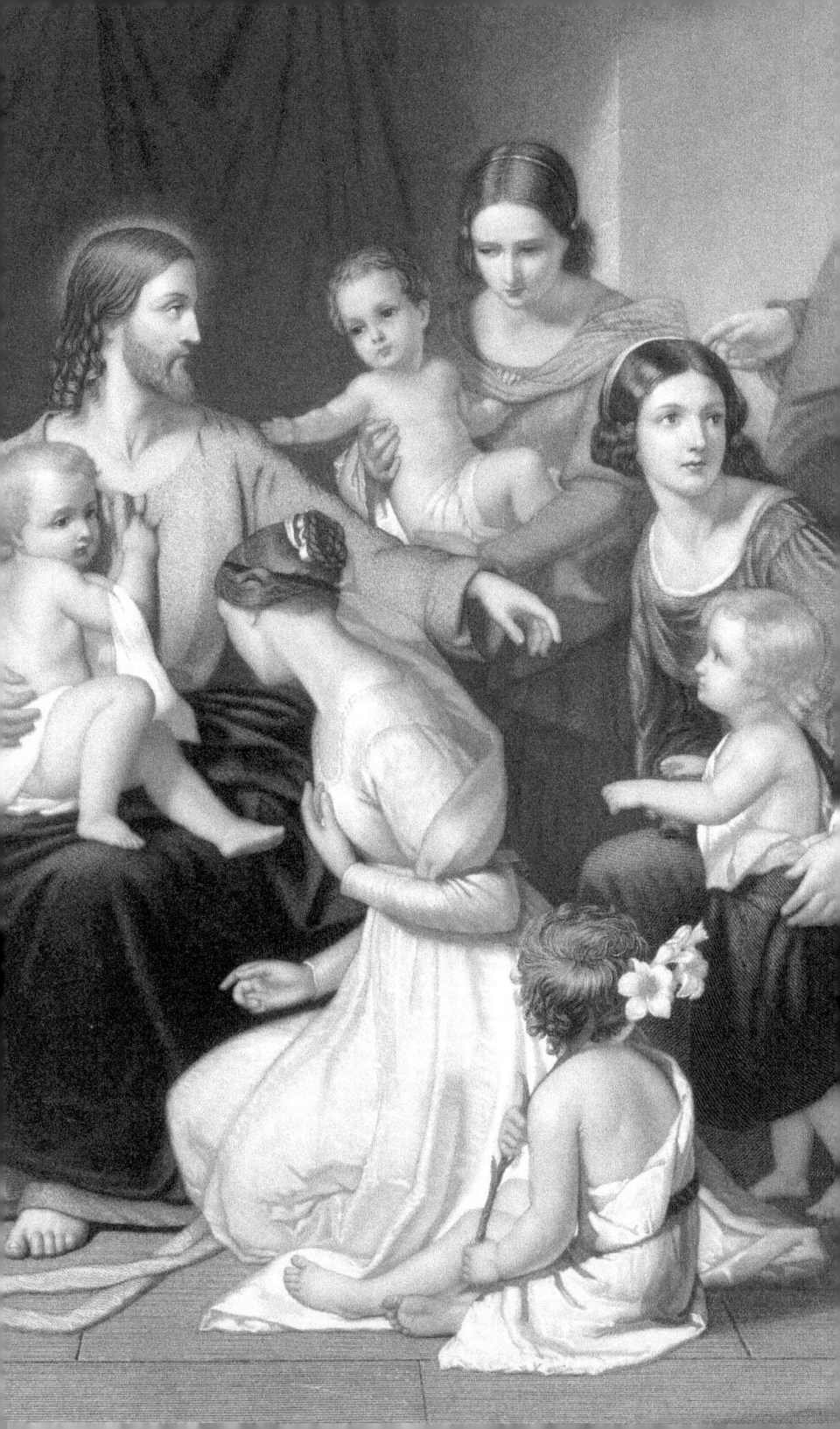

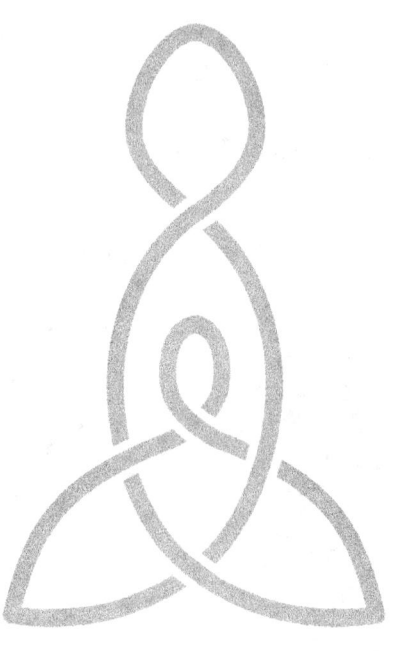